Praise for *Losing Sight, Finding Vision: Thriving Throughout Life's Lasting Losses*

Follow Sheridan's journey in *Losing Sight, Finding Vision*, and you will gain insights into the power of meditation, self-reflection, and listening to the wisdom of the body when dealing with any of life's challenges. This book is a beautiful illustration of how we can respond to long-term loss and discover the courage and wisdom of our own heart.
—Tara Brach, Ph.D., Author of *Radical Acceptance* and *True Refuge*

Losing Sight, Finding Vision is a remarkable story of courage, commitment, and the enduring power of compassion. Sheridan Gates' vision of leadership and transformation is intimate and far reaching. There are gems here that enlighten one's professional life as well as enriching the heart.
—Richard Strozzi-Heckler, Ph.D.
Author of *The Art of Somatic Coaching* and *The Leadership Dojo*

Sheridan Gates has written a wonderful book describing her journey with vision loss, which serves as a much-needed primer for others facing similar challenges. This book is also a must-read for family members who have a loved one that is experiencing chronic vision loss. Sheridan has captured the innermost feelings and emotions a visually impaired person might be going through but will not always be able to express in such eloquent words.

Losing Sight, Finding Vision serves as an inspiration for others who are traveling a similar journey of adapting to loss. Thank you for writing this book.
—Suleiman Alibhai, O.D.

Losing Sight, Finding Vision lights the way to living fully rather than getting caught in anxiety about the inevitable losses of life, health, and loved ones. Taking us on an honest walk through her vision loss, Sheridan Gates is like a good friend, reminding us of our resourcefulness and potential.

—Klia Bassing, MBA, MPP, founder of VisitYourself.net and author of @visityourself on Twitter

Losing Sight, Finding Vision will open readers' eyes to the spirit and strengths within. This engaging book is an inspirational read that applies to many life challenges. I appreciated the insights that Sheridan shared with her readers. I would recommend this book to anyone facing challenges related to their health, along with their families and friends.

Readers gain insights into practical strategies such as meditation, self-reflection, and listening to the wisdom of the body as Sheridan applies these in her own journey.

—Michele Hartlove, Executive Director, Prevention of Blindness Society

Sheridan Gates' spectacular reframing of the vision loss of macular degeneration into the deep wisdom of insight is nothing short of an inspiration to us all. Her vivid inner journey challenges readers to take the risk of opening up their greater awareness and expanding their connection to life itself!

—Desda Zuckerman, author of *Your Sacred Anatomy: An Owner's Guide to the Human Energy Structure*, and founder of CoreIndividuation™

In *Losing Sight, Finding Vision*, Sheridan Gates tells her story with honesty, courage, and authenticity.

The story alone provides guidance for others on a similar journey, but Sheridan's reflections and invitations offer additional concrete healing possibilities.

As a Pastoral Counselor and Spiritual Director, I am grateful to have such a tool to suggest to clients.

—Charlotte Rogers, LPC

In *Losing Sight, Finding Vision*, Sheridan Gates deftly weaves the story of her own vision loss with the skills and techniques of spiritual sight gained as she copes with her challenges. Her perceptive questions and practical suggestions will help anyone develop their inner seeing and knowing. In my lines of work, I have learned this is the most important vision of all.

—The Rev. Ann Gillespie,
Episcopal priest and yoga teacher

If you are looking for a way through loss to thriving, read this book. Sheridan Gates is an exemplar of what it means to walk your talk. In her book *Losing Sight, Finding Vision* she shares that walk with candor and openness. She offers sign posts along the path so we can all find a way through life's greatest challenges with dignity, grace and fullness in the face of anything.

—Jennifer L. Cohen
Seven Stones Leadership Group

Losing Sight, Finding Vision

Thriving Throughout Life's Lasting Losses

Sheridan Gates

Copyright © 2014 Purpose At Work

ALL RIGHTS RESERVED

No part of this book may be translated, used, or reproduced in any form or by any means, in whole or in part, electronic or mechanical, including photocopying, recording, taping, or by any information storage or retrieval system without express written permission from the author or the publisher, except for the use in brief quotations within critical articles and reviews.

(Sheridan@purposeatwork.com www.losingsightfindingvision.com)

Limits of Liability and Disclaimer of Warranty:

The authors and/or publisher shall not be liable for your misuse of this material. The contents are strictly for informational and educational purposes only.

Warning—Disclaimer:

The purpose of this book is to educate and entertain. The authors and/or publisher do not guarantee that anyone following these techniques, suggestions, tips, ideas, or strategies will become successful. The author and/or publisher shall have neither liability nor responsibility to anyone with respect to any loss or damage caused, or alleged to be caused, directly or indirectly by the information contained in this book. Further, readers should be aware that Internet websites listed in this work may have changed or disappeared between when this work was written and when it is read.

Printed and bound in the United States of America
ISBN: 978-0-692-22616-2
Library of Congress Control Number: 2014910221

Dedication

To my mother, whose way of seeing the world creates both love and possibilities.

Acknowledgments

This book reflects 30 years of living and learning. I am very grateful to those who have accompanied me on this journey from the early stages of resisting unwanted change to thriving. From those who've shared their own journey with similar challenges, to those whom I've supported, I'm so grateful to travel this path with so many courageous souls.

To the many people who encouraged me in this creative process, friends, family, and fellow writers, I so appreciate the wisdom and help I've received. I offer thanks to M. J. Ryan, Frank Steele, Bethany Kelly, Karma Bennet and Nancy Shanteau, whose professional writing and publishing experience helped me bring this book into the world.

To the many teachers who have taught me about living fully, being a coach and a healer—Tara Brach, Richard Strozzi-Heckler, Julio Olalla, and Desda Zuckerman.

Table of Contents

Introduction 1
Chapter 1: Being with Your Experience 4
Chapter 2: Seeing Your Wholeness.. 19
Chapter 3: Accessing Dignity 37
Chapter 4: Orienting from Purpose.. 52
Chapter 5: Cultivating Embodied Wisdom 75
Chapter 6: Navigating from Within... 94
Chapter 7: Living from the Core 108
Chapter 8: Honoring Yourself as You Learn 124
Chapter 9: Connecting Authentically with Others 139
Chapter 10: Expanding Your Aperture 153
Notes... 168
Resources 174
Recommended books 175
About the Author 178

Introduction

When I first read the phrase "finding the wellness within the illness" in "Successful and Schizophrenic" by Elyn R. Saks in the *New York Times*, I smiled.[1] Saks, a law professor at the University of Southern California and author of the memoir *The Center Cannot Hold: My Journey Through Madness*, distilled those factors which most contributed to success for those with schizophrenia.[2] One study participant suggested finding wellness in the illness should be the therapeutic goal for all those diagnosed with schizophrenia.

Not just schizophrenia, I thought to myself. For over 30 years, I have been on a journey toward thriving as I adjust to juvenile macular degeneration. And for the past two years, I have captured this very sentiment in a book that was taking shape. But when it came to thinking of myself as ill, I squirmed. I realized that I don't see myself as ill. And as I thought about others whose lives inspired me as they faced illness or disability, I cringed when I thought of them as ill. To me, they were inspiring heroes and heroines who embodied courage and aliveness.

In a conversation with my friend Barbara, who also lives with vision impairment, I ask her, "What enables you to thrive?" She balks at the notion that her illness enables courage or strengths to emerge. She says, "I cannot separate out the illness as a distinct influence in my life." She feels she is simply living her life—and that her many strengths are part of the natural evolution of her maturation and development as a human being. How could she attribute her gifts directly or indirectly to her experience of sight loss?

Barbara mentions something I'd noticed but had not considered before: the internal impulse to thrive results in courage. Others who witness this courage and commitment to living fully often become inspired and motivated to thrive themselves. What we describe as courage is simply the individual responding from his or her internal inner web of values, gifts, and convictions, like the Paralympic athlete who is simply following the impulse to excel.

We all know people who demonstrate courage and a spirit of thriving despite illness or adversity. We admire their creativity and aliveness. We wonder if we can exhibit such admirable qualities when we face our own challenges. I am here to say that it is indeed quite possible. That's what this book is all about.

In *Losing Sight, Finding Vision* I share my discoveries regarding how to forge a path of dignity, authenticity, and meaning while adjusting to long-term illness or life-altering challenges. If you have low vision and are looking for a book that prescribes everyday fixes to accommodate vision loss, you will be disappointed. If you want to explore how to thrive so you can forge an authentic response to loss and change, this book is for you.

In my own journey with sight loss, my inner sight awakened. Seeing myself as a whole person and not as someone with vision impairment has given me a sense of dignity in the face of loss. Seeing the gifts and possibilities in others has enabled me to serve as a coach and a healer. Seeing the brilliance in life's unfolding has enabled a sense of serenity and trust in me as I have encountered challenges. Recasting challenges as opportunities to innovate has reframed loss into transformation.

In this book I offer lessons on what it means to thrive while living with a life-altering challenge or illness. As my friend suggests, enabling our learning and development to prevail as we navigate through loss and change fosters dignity.

INTRODUCTION

I introduce ten strategies which emerged over my three decades of gradual sight loss. These strategies resulted from trial and error. As I bungled through, reacting to unwanted changes, I discovered what I could do to foster well-being.

For each of the ten strategies I highlight both practical and soul-enhancing ways to access our full aliveness. I invite you to engage in your own inquiry—"What would fully thriving look like for me?"—as you read each chapter.

Living solely based on others' expectations or our prognosis thwarts our sense of aliveness. We may not be able to change our diagnosis, but we can change our experience and perhaps our prognosis. As we consider the fullness of our soul and spirit, not just the diagnosis or adversity, we recognize the many choices which foster wellness and wholeness in our lives. Join me on this journey to intentionally deepen fulfillment and vitality in your life as you discover the wellness and wholeness within.

CHAPTER 1

BEING WITH YOUR EXPERIENCE

"Sometimes our light goes out but is blown again into flame by an encounter with another human being. Each of us owes the deepest thanks to those who have rekindled this inner light."

—Albert Schweitzer

WASHINGTON DC, 1988. As my workday draws to a close, I motor into the hectic Washington Beltway rush hour. My vision is nearly 20/200: legal blindness according to the DMV. I have difficulty seeing what is directly in front of me.

I trail an endless line of vehicles amid six lanes of traffic. Cars move at widely varying speeds, weaving from lane to lane. Fatigue lulls my senses as I drift toward the end of a long day. I picture arriving home, changing out of this business suit, and heating up a TV dinner.

Out of nowhere glaring brake lights flash directly in front of me. It was as if the car came through some imaginary screen in an instant. One second, no car, the next second, brake lights within crash distance.

I swerve over to the right lane. My heart races. I gasp for breath. As I continue down the highway at 65 miles per hour, the moment reverberates throughout my body. A burst of adrenaline sends shock waves to my limbs. I feel my severe sight loss like a bolt of lightning.

I've been ignoring this huge change in my physical abilities, hoping if I just tried hard enough, it would not affect my life or livelihood. I've narrowly escaped a rear-end collision. I grip the steering wheel like I cling to my memory of a world in which I have full sight. The mix of intense fear, shame, denial, and sheer bewilderment swirls within me like some slow-cooking stew on a hot stove. I can no longer drive safely.

However, driving is essential to my work. I traverse a four-state territory marketing my company's family of mutual funds to investment advisors. My strongest impulse is to hold on to my job.

I acquire the ability to navigate with limited vision while behind the steering wheel. Occasionally I approach an intersection without knowing whether the light is red or green. I rely on movements of nearby cars to serve as proxies for the traffic light. It's like being at the edge of a cliff and just plain not seeing a way forward. It takes months before I tell my employer I can no longer drive.

Looking back, I cringe at how I placed my own and others' lives in jeopardy. It was only a matter of time before I caused a car accident. But I was so identified with my work that I couldn't imagine a future without it.

Loss, Loss, and More Loss

In 1982 I am diagnosed with the juvenile form of macular degeneration called Stargardt's disease. It is an inherited and progressive disease, but not altogether blinding. It affects the pinpoint center of the retina, the macula, and affects straightforward central vision.

At this time I do not think of myself as someone on a learning journey around seeing. Like many folks in their early 20s, I have ambitions to find true love and rise in my profession. At a more surface level, my goals include finding the best appetizers at downtown Chicago happy hours, affordably decorating my tiny 500-square-foot apartment, and losing the proverbial 10 pounds. Life seems full of possibilities and opportunities to learn, acquire, and become.

Upon first learning of my diagnosis, I rely heavily on denial and avoidance. I hear that when I am 40, I may no longer be able to drive. As a young and hopeful Chicagoan, this means little to me as long as I can catch the 156 LaSalle bus downtown for work. I mostly store this information in some invisible corner of my mind and go about my life.

Facing the Loss

A few months after my near collision on the Beltway, someone tells me it is one thing to face lifelong vision loss, but another to cause a serious traffic accident. The comparison crystallizes my situation in a way that I have not understood until now. What am I thinking? Is my job worth risking my life, not to mention others' lives? Holding on to my job so tightly is blinding me to the risks and consequences of driving with vision impairment. How could I not have seen this?

Not being able to drive means I need to leave my current position. The office manager begins searching for a replacement. I apply for disability leave. I explore some positions within the firm that would not require me to drive, but they are not a fit for me. What I love about my job is training and coaching investment professionals in estate planning strategies using our mutual fund product. Something in me wants to move on, even though I don't know why.

During my last weeks at the firm, I work with the woman who will be taking my job. We spend time in the office as I share with her the systems and organization I've created. We travel to introduce her to the leading companies I had worked with to facilitate the transition. In those hand-off meetings I awkwardly joke that I am retiring, a prospect that frankly feels too close to the truth.

Other than a three-week vacation, I have no real plans. I certainly do not know what I'll do next in terms of career, let alone what I'll do with my time. I feel like a bumbling log headed for a dramatic drop down a waterfall just beyond my view. I don't know what to expect, but I can't imagine that it will be good.

The complaints I had been airing about my job diminish as feelings of loss emerge. So many good people, so great to share my expertise with others who are eager to learn, so much freedom to accomplish goals as I see fit.

This time in between one chapter of my life and another feels surreal. I amble through each step without much thought about what is ahead. Each day seems more alive than usual, as I know the days are dwindling. The allure of some ideal future slips away as my final workday draws near.

I bet you are reading this book because in some way you are on a journey similar to mine. Something has happened to knock you off the path you thought you were taking and onto new, uncomfortable, or even painful and terrifying terrain. I want to offer you a hand in the darkness, footsteps to follow. I write not so much as an expert, but as someone who has been on this journey to find the wellness in my illness for nearly 30 years. As a result, I've developed a set of ten strategies I've found helpful for myself. I've also gathered good advice from others in similar circumstances. Together these strategies may give you a sense of resilience while you navigate through change and loss.

I've come a long way since I drove recklessly because of my fear of what was happening to me. But I keenly remember what it feels like to be in that place, and I want you to know you are not alone. I hope this book will help you to tap into your strengths and cultivate a sense of thriving.

So Many Questions

As I approach the last day on my job, I focus my energy on planning my "retirement trip"—a three-week adventure from Hawaii to Australia. After the trip, now on disability, I return to the questions that are staring at me: At 29, what am I going to do with the rest of my life? Will I ever work again? Will anyone hire me?

My fears and concerns are both near- and long-term. If my vision is already 20/200, what will my visual acuity be at age 40 and beyond? How will I read if my vision deteriorates further? What will a life without driving be like and what options will this preclude? I imagine myself at 40, wearing dark glasses as I hold tightly to the leash of my German Shepherd guide dog, stumbling over furniture in my apartment, lonely and without resources.

I feel as if I am flailing without a rudder amid a stormy sea, being tossed and whipped about. In some ways, I don't want to know the answers to these questions. I don't possess an emotional buffer or safety net large enough to contain my anxieties. Nor do I know anyone who has already traversed this unexpected detour so early in life. The sense of helplessness and fear pervades my daily life.

I explore new age spiritual texts to find a source of solace and comfort. The idea that we create our own reality offers promise and possibility. While these teachings help me begin to develop self-awareness and personal power, they make me feel as if I am to blame for my eye condition.

The popular refrain I keep hearing is, "Why don't you want to see?" Or "What do you not want to see?" "What happened at the time of your vision loss that you were avoiding?" The creative interpretations of disease offered by such thinkers as Louise Hay send me into an inward lament. Ultimately it comes down to: "What did I do to cause this disease?"

Blaming myself for what happened seems wrong. It only makes things more difficult. I don't know what to think or how to proceed. Mostly I grasp for ways to avoid my pain. I want immediate relief from my sense of loss and fear rather than a deep and lasting spiritual awakening. This spiritual yearning feels desperate and compulsive, rather than peaceful.

I work to change my thoughts with an iron fist. I do not feel capable of creating calm through this spiritual quest, which feels more like an obsession to me. I alternate between doing affirmations like, "I now see perfectly," reading metaphysical writings, and working to forgive past hurts and disappointments. Anxiety is a core driver. I wallow in self-pity and doubt.

Looking back now, I see I didn't allow myself space to grieve because I felt so afraid that if I met my grief head-on, it would envelop me entirely.

Metabolizing Disappointment

During this time of adjustment, a career counselor explains the stages of loss to me from the Elisabeth Kübler-Ross (EKR) grief cycle. This cycle is a natural emotional reaction to trauma and personal change, not just death and dying. Transitions between stages in the cycle can occur more like ebb and flow rather than a linear progression.[1] This explains why some days I feel hopeful and other days I feel discouraged. It helps me to have more compassion for myself, for my inability to grasp reality all in one chunk. Not only am I dealing with the loss of my sight, but also of my career.

One of the challenges with macular degeneration is the progressive nature of the disease. One eye-care professional tells me that about every ten years I will encounter enough vision loss that I will have to change the way I do certain things. In *On Death and Dying,* Elisabeth Kübler-Ross defines the grieving process in terms of what is now six stages.² Imagine moving through these phases every ten years or so.

- ▶ Denial/Shock
- ▶ Anger
- ▶ Bargaining
- ▶ Depression
- ▶ Testing/Experimentation
- ▶ Acceptance

Denial

As I reflect, downplaying my experience of vision loss helped me move through grief in waves. Early in my sight-loss journey, apart from changing my eyeglasses, I operated as if nothing had changed. If my vision didn't prevent me from doing something, why not do it?

Minimizing my limitations enabled me to stretch and grow. I wasn't able to drive, but I could read, bike, play tennis, hike, and knit, and so my life seemed unchanged in many ways. As long as I could do something I enjoyed, I did it. And somehow this fact emboldened me to pretend my future would be different than doctors foretold.

As I explored career options, I imagined that I could reinvent my career without constraints. I gave some thought to the progressive vision loss that lay ahead, but almost defiantly pushed it aside. Becoming a pilot or a brain surgeon didn't appeal to me anyway! Severe vision loss seemed years away. I was determined to neither be defined by nor identified with my eye disease.

My pace quickens. I jump at the opportunities to connect with others, for I feel very alone. I join a group beach house during the summers and find myself newly addicted to activity. If I move fast enough, maybe it won't feel so bad, my thinking goes.

Anger

My habitual ways of experiencing anger include blame, perfectionism, and resentment. When the HR manager notified me that my long-term disability claim had been approved, I felt angry toward him, as if he'd taken away my job. I felt as though I'd been fired. I was angry at the company for not serving up an ideal job option for me. I had been such a devoted employee—how could they let me go? I felt as if I were being pushed aside at the peak of my career while my peers were on the rise.

And now my professional relationships dwindle as I disconnect from the firm. My experience seems so abrupt, even though several months have gone by since I first told my boss I could no longer drive.

Every unconscious negative belief I have finds new life in my present circumstances. Rounds of "Things never work out for me" serenade inside me as I go to sleep each night. I awaken at 2:00 a.m. to the tune of "There must be something wrong with me," which permeates my rattled mind until dawn. The more I give in to this negative thinking, the more it drenches my life with darkened prospects for my future. I keep playing these tapes over and over again in my head.

I can't seem to fix my gaze toward my future. I feel reactive for months. Instead of paying attention to my internal experience and feelings, I continue to fight with the realities I face. I leap into spiritual fellowships in a desperate attempt to find a sense of belonging. Yet my deep vulnerability and mistrust catch up with me again and again, as I feel disappointed by others, by life, by the way things keep turning out.

My anger also lashes out at others. I am impatient with clerks, customer service representatives, and anyone who disappoints me. Is it so hard to just do what I ask them to do? And underneath this anger, I am truly lost and afraid. My dreams for my future are slipping away and some new unwelcome reality is bubbling to the surface. Surely I will never be able to feel a sense of possibility and hope again. I had the courage to tell my employer I could no longer drive, but do I really possess the strength to live out the consequences of this action?

Bargaining

It may be hard to believe that anyone experiencing vision loss could possibly question the reality of impaired vision. You'd be surprised. The words *incurable* and *irreversible* are just concepts. Even the realities of sight loss seem as if they can be overcome by the human spirit. The desire to triumph over adversity, the power of hope, and the allure of faith play significant roles in shaping my perspective: "Maybe *my* experience of macular degeneration will be different." What if I can cure it through alternative healing therapies?

One doctor tells me of a study conducted in the lab with mice. The mice were injected with the same type of diseased cells as those in my retina. One group of mice was kept in the dark, with no exposure to light. The other group was regularly exposed to light. Over the course of the study, the mice without light exposure did not experience sight loss. The mice exposed to light experienced the same gradual visual loss as me.[3]

The doctor urges me to avoid overexposure to direct sunlight. The use of protective sunglasses and a hat during summer months are recommended as preventive measures to protect my eyes. I vow to wear the sunglasses and hat, yet I make a conscious choice not to avoid being outdoors. I love hiking, biking, and walking in nature. Maybe I will scale down my beach time, but I cannot imagine my life without the outdoors. Who wants to hang out with a mole anyway?

While these choices help me feel in charge of my life, every time I gloss over the sharp edges of impending loss, I feel even more vulnerable to the changes I face. Negotiating with my diagnosis by assuming alternative therapies will cure my condition distracts me from accepting reality.

Depression

One interpretation of depression is acceptance without detachment. It's as if the wound of my vision loss is raw and exposed. The wound festers, and the balm or healing ointment doesn't relieve the pain. It's difficult to imagine healing or change.

I realize that having a stable work network provided a needed social context and helped me feel connected. Without this, I feel isolated, as I face uncertainty both about my vision and my future. I seem to connect less and less with my work peers. This is my most profound experience of loneliness to date. It's as though I'm an iceberg which has broken away from a glacier, wandering out to sea, with the connectedness appearing farther away with each glance.

I've also learned that depression is anger turned inward. I blame myself in some unconscious way for this abrupt loss. I wonder if I can parent, travel alone, and even continue to appreciate beauty in nature. Facing a life of continual decline can only happen to someone who deserves it, right? Am I too selfish? What did I do to deserve this? I grew up driving, born in the suburbs into a family that owned a car dealership, no less, and I can no longer drive? So I can't live in the suburbs or fulfill my childhood fantasy of living on a farm.

Testing and Experimentation

I consult a low-vision specialist and purchase aids to facilitate my daily activities. I begin carrying in my purse a small handheld magnifier to read small print on items like price tags. I invest $3,000 in a video magnifier to read larger blocks of text, including magazines and books. I purchase a voice memo recorder to capture grocery lists and to-do items. Leveraging my current vision becomes my goal.

My low-vision specialist recommends I attend nearby support groups to meet others with similar challenges. At first I avoid these groups as if they are contagious. Then I reluctantly check out a few groups. I feel uneasy when I meet someone using a cane. Will that be me in 10 years? 20 years? I can barely face my future.

Slowly I learn more about this new world of coping with vision loss. I make a few friends as I drop in to the various blindness communities and become open to learning from their experience. I become a mass transit frequent rider and explore outlying stations.

Somewhere in this transition between the loss of my work and my new life as a person with low vision, I begin to *want* to thrive. I want what is happening to me to fit into some larger context that will help me to make sense of life as I am coming to know it. I hunger for a greater meaning or purpose to it all. Conversations with friends and spiritual seekers and teachers help me to cultivate this yearning.

I toggle between denial, depression, and acceptance, just as the EKR grief cycle describes. Every time I think I've accepted my vision loss, another wave of disappointment sweeps through me. Eye exams, an encounter with someone who doesn't understand my challenge, or a last-minute sprint through an airport resurrects feelings of anxiety or frustration. The very basic nature of my challenge serves as a humbling equalizer. Activities that I once took for granted now activate my vulnerability. I hesitate when I enter a dimly lit elevator. Which button do I push?

I have a quest, albeit possibly a compulsion, to fix, to heal my eyes. I am much more interested in healing than in accepting the loss. I'm not sure if my quest is simply the normal garden-variety lack of acceptance or bargaining that accompanies a loss like mine, or whether it's unique in some way. The question I ponder is how to face the realities, the medical knowledge and known limitations linked to my eye disease, and how to find hope for healing.

As I move between these two points of view, I bump into each awkwardly, always forgetting that my vision is not supposed to get better, only worse. Then I get disappointed all over again. I want to heal, not be continually disappointed by my daily realities.

As I wander through the experience of loss, weaving together lessons from others and myself, I yearn for a compass to guide me. Rather than try to change the unchangeable, my deteriorating vision, perhaps I can steady myself in some other way. The disorientation of blurred vision jars my nervous system, and the constant adjustment to gradual loss continually pushes me outside my comfort zone. I need an inner compass, because without it, the pain and loss are too great.

Acceptance

When I fully embrace the current realities, I experience a settling in my nervous system. I no longer need things to be different in order to be at ease. I stop trying to manage my inner experiences or my outer circumstances. A new sense of ease permeates my inner landscape and steadies my mood.

Low-vision specialists, counselors, fellow seekers, and others with vision loss help me to reach this place. Each caring conversation inches me toward acceptance. I learn again and again that I am not alone, and the compassion I receive strengthens my self-acceptance. Soon I can pass along my own lessons to others facing a fresh diagnosis of macular degeneration. I begin to see myself as connected in so many ways, and my personal loss transmutes into a well-worn notch in the tree of my life.

Being with Our Experiences

The first strategy for thriving involves truly being present for our direct experiences. When a threat to our life as we know it looms, we all experience the emotional cycle described in the EKR grief model. We each move through this cycle at our own pace, but ultimately we're forced to face the reality that the assumptions that so neatly held our life together are not as solid as we first thought. There is a breaking apart that happens inside when we realize this.

Facing the truth of our circumstances enables us to deal with them. I remember hearing somewhere that letting go is really just accepting the truth of what is happening. As we become willing to meet our life circumstances honestly, we slowly begin to feel less anxious, less afraid. As we pay attention to our own experience of change and loss, our feelings, the sensations in our bodies, and our own thinking, we befriend ourselves. This is being with ourselves. Although nothing changes, we become open to possibilities. It happened to me, and it can happen to you too.

Even if we can only swallow a small dose of our reality at a time, a sense of dignity accompanies this turning toward the truth. We begin to accept our lives more fully as they are and stop rejecting ourselves and our experiences.

As we move toward and not away from our circumstances, we build the skill to remain curious about our difficult experiences. We begin to notice what it is like from the inside out. We pay attention to what we are feeling and sensing.

Being present for our experience means seeing clearly, without the heavy fog of denial and depression. When we do see clearly, we open ourselves up to the possibility that acceptance will replace feelings of disappointment and discouragement. We can't force this process, nor how much reality we can metabolize in any given day. But as we move toward this place, we can begin to shape our way of accepting what is happening, to have a sense that we can make a difference in our own lives.

To help you reach that place, I encourage you to connect with others who face similar challenges. The friends and family who surrounded me before this journey were often unable to relate to my experiences. But I became energized when I engaged with others facing the same diagnosis.

When I had conversations with such people, I shifted from feeling like a victim into the realization that I was not alone. As I shared some piece of wisdom with another, I contributed to others and recognized that I still have value.

While this process can't be forced and each person's journey is unique, there are some ways to help yourself learn to be engaged in your direct experience. Start by being honest with yourself about your situation. Ask, "What changes are on the horizon and what will this mean for me?" Listen inwardly for what is really important for you as you experience these changes. Keep track of your emotional climate as you adapt to the loss or change you face. View your emotions as natural expressions of change, meeting difficult feelings directly with kindness. Connect with others facing similar challenges and find ways to gain perspective. When you are ready, experiment by paying close attention to your thoughts and feelings and sharing these with others to help you adapt to your new life.

QUESTION

What conversations—both inside you and with others—are increasing your energy and possibilities?

Practice

> How are you talking about what's going on for you to the people in your life? Stretch yourself to share with others what you are facing. Share with those who have similar experiences. Practice being real about what is happening, being witnessed by those whom you trust.

CHAPTER 2

SEEING YOUR WHOLENESS

"I see my life as an unfolding set of opportunities to awaken."
—Ram Dass

At a young age, I longed to join the working world. So at the age of 14, I started working at my first real job—as a server at a nearby Baskin-Robbins ice cream store. This job afforded me the indulgence of two true loves—connecting with people and food. Sporting my "shocking pink" uniform and my best smile, I taste-tested, dipped and wrapped cones, offered tasty samples, and moved about the store with pride and joy.

One of the many benefits was a free treat for the family member who picked me up after closing. I remember how proudly I deposited my paychecks into my passbook savings account and recorded the amount in my checkbook ledger. It didn't matter to me then that I was only making $1.10 an hour; what mattered was that I was establishing autonomy and developing a taste for financial independence. I could buy the clothes I wanted without asking for money from my mom. I could save up for things that mattered to me and not depend solely on my allowance or birthday checks from my grandmother.

In my many forms of work over the years, I've always resonated with the virtues of autonomy and financial independence. As a young girl in the

1970s, I sensed that this basic right to work was integral to self-respect and freedom. Episodes of the *Mary Tyler Moore Show* shaped my young but ambitious mind. I admired the autonomy my parents possessed in their respective careers. I wanted that level of independence and power and saw a career as the way to achieve it. If I could carve out a successful path for myself, I could pave the way to a bright future. This future could steady me in the face of life's unpredictable nature.

These values probably explain why the bedrock within me shook so deeply when I elected to go on long-term disability at 29. My fears about my ability to earn an income in the future converged with my fears about losing my vision. The two fears painted a dark picture. I couldn't imagine another employer hiring me. I had transferred to Washington DC for my job and now felt lost.

Would I ever work again? What would become of me? I saw no models around me of others who had traveled this particular journey. My fears painted such a vivid picture, disregarding all the virtues of my hard-work ethic, the goodwill of others, or the possibilities that I could not yet see.

Are you experiencing this kind of fear and feeling overwhelmed? Has fear collapsed or distorted your sense of a situation to the point where you no longer consider the possibilities? In this chapter we will explore moving through fear and accessing our strengths. Because it is only when we see our wholeness that we can have the courage to change the things we can.

Seeing our wholeness enables us to live life fully—accessing our power and advocating for ourselves when necessary. Seeing ourselves as whole takes the sting out of identifying with our illness, or seeing our challenge as the defining influence in our path through life. Dignity and self-respect accompany us daily as we make choices in our lives that honor our wholeness.

Designing the Future

Once I return from my "retirement" trip to Australia, I pick up Richard Bolles' book, *What Color is Your Parachute?*, work through the exercises, and begin to see some patterns.[1] I love teaching, helping, and connecting with others. I begin informational interviewing to see what possible career options might work for me.

The picture is very hazy for some time. I pursue all kinds of ideas, from becoming a travel agent to going to graduate school. I am one of those people who really benefit from career books, workshops, and counseling. I get lost in possibilities pretty easily and have trouble making decisions, which for me means cutting off possibilities. Putting a stake in the ground and discerning which path to pursue too early in my exploratory process is like poking a hole in my "possibility balloon" before I finish inflating it.

The core interests and skills that emerge from this inquiry are training, facilitation, and adult learning. A year or so into my time on long-term disability, I start graduate school at George Washington University. The School of Education has a master's degree in human development with an emphasis on training design.

I dip my toe in the water by taking one course, then another, until I connect to a wave of inner enthusiasm and can see a possible career future. I decide to hone my skills designing and delivering training to become a trainer and consultant in organizational learning and development.

Halfway through graduate school, I receive a job offer from a company in Boston. I feel tension as I consider this opportunity, typical of big decisions at this time. As part of my extroverted nature, I gather input from several sources—family members, friends, professional colleagues—and then become confused by the divergence of opinions. Some say it's best to take the job, even if it means a move. Others recognize my ambivalence about moving.

I schedule an appointment with a spiritual director at the Institute for Attitudinal Healing, where I attend classes on the Course in Miracles.[2] In our meeting, I summarize the key elements of the situation and feel deeply heard by her as she leads me through the process. I take a breath and ask, "What do you think?"

She says, "I notice that when you talk about Boston, there is a background of fear, concern, anxiety, and worry. When you talk about staying in Washington, there is a sense of peace and ease." She pauses and I let her words sink in. My whole body relaxes.

"I do feel uneasy about uprooting myself right now," I acknowledge. "Years ago, I would have loved to move to Boston. But now, it just feels hard."

She continues, "The Course in Miracles encourages us to make decisions based on love, not fear. In your case, your fears and concerns seem greatest when you speak about moving."

I answer, "Yes, the fear seems very real. Some part of me also feels like it is crazy not to take a job offer when I don't have a job."

"Tell me more about the sense of peace," she says.

"I never thought I'd stay in Washington more than a few years, but it's come to feel like home. I don't really want to let all that go."

She recommends that I choose based on peace rather than fear. This means letting go of the internal pressure to take the job due to fear I won't find another one that is a better fit. Choosing in this way is a novel and profound idea for me. It means turning inward for my authority.

I turn down the job offer and start my next semester in school with a full load of courses. Looking back, this was not just a career decision. It was the first time I made a choice that was in alignment with my inner sense of wisdom and peace. It set the course for a new paradigm which called me to live more fully from that which enlivened me personally, regardless of others' opinions. It was a step toward activating my own heroine's journey.

Landing

I develop friendships with classmates. I join the local chapter of the American Society for Training and Development and meet people who work in the field of adult learning. Slowly I begin to see myself in this new profession. I become an intern for an independent consultant. Under her guidance I develop training materials for her work with the government. On one occasion I deliver a portion of training for one of her clients. I begin networking in search of a full-time job.

Toward the end of my graduate studies, I take a job with a large management consulting firm. The work and study I had done in leadership development and quality improvement fit into the federal Quality and Change Management practice of the local office. How perfect for someone who is undergoing so much change at a personal level!

I spend my first year supporting the development of the firm's Center of Excellence for Quality. In addition to doing some client work developing leadership training, I draft marketing materials, coordinate a firm-wide partner meeting on quality, and edit an internal newsletter.

While on the surface I'm succeeding, at some deep level, mostly invisible to me, I feel damaged. I see myself as much more vulnerable, like a bird with a broken wing. I internalize this sense of "not okay-ness" and presume this is how others see me. Even though I interviewed for this job with a sense of hope for a more solid career future, I now hold corrosive thoughts like: *I have to accept what's given to me because I am not fully-abled. It's my fault if something doesn't work out.*

I carry this underlying self-doubt into my new work environment. On difficult projects I push myself because I feel I have to be without blemish. I feel as if the implicit contract I'm making is that I have to be so flawless and dedicated that I am beyond being let go. Still reeling from my last abrupt job loss, I strive to hold tightly to my employer as a way of securing my future.

So I work hard, very hard. I lead the development and delivery of an experiential leadership training program for a government agency client. The top leaders have embraced participative management and want the top 300 leaders to develop this style more fully.

I lead the design of a new course without any existing course material. I have a team of folks who support me in the many details of this project. I begin to see the complexities of organizational change and to recognize the limitations of training as a stand-alone solution to large-scale systems change. We implement several supportive processes, such as updating the agency's leadership performance measures to reflect the desired change.

Serving as a facilitator to teams, I witness the power of shared purpose in building commitment and action. Working with teams to move through stumbling blocks is both challenging and fulfilling. I work with a government agency team focusing on improving a highly visible administrative process. One of their challenges is "analysis paralysis." As a group of analytical people, they keep getting bogged down in conversation. I mirror back to the group what I am seeing, and they begin to laugh at themselves.

They amend their group norms to include keeping focused and avoiding beating a dead horse. The next meeting I bring in a plastic toy horse, a relic from my childhood. They take to tapping the horse with the side of a pen to give real-time feedback to a team member who is waxing on too long about something that is no longer relevant or useful.

As my vision deteriorates, I overcompensate for my vision loss. I memorize overheads and conceal my loss from clients. In a culture where competition is alive and perfectionism is rewarded, it seems appropriate. Then one day, a partner calls me into his office and tells me a client contacted him because she notices my eyes aren't squarely looking at her during a training meeting.

When I look at someone, my eyes compensate for my blind spot by looking to the side slightly. It's noticeable to others, and can cause some confusion. I notice people often looking behind them when facing me, wondering if I'm looking at them or someone else.

I feel ashamed, as if I have let somebody down. In actuality, the client wants to encourage me to disclose my visual challenges. She thinks it will help me to avoid misunderstanding during training. Rather than pretend I don't have this challenge, she feels I need to take the risk and expose my vulnerability. She's right.

I begin disclosing my eye challenge, trying to maintain my professionalism and dignity when I share this personal information. Frequently people come up at the break and share challenges they are experiencing, as a way of building connection with me. Folks comment that I seem to do so well given that I see less than 10 percent of what most people see. It's as if my colleagues and clients are giving me a pat on the back for not standing out or struggling with my vision. This is a very mixed message.

On the one hand, it's a negative compliment. I take comments such as these as a sign that if I can continue to minimize my challenge, everyone will value me more. If I hide my vision challenges and perform just like others, I will not pose any awkwardness for others or myself.

On the other hand, such comments imply an affirmation. People are resonating with my confidence and strengths. Many colleagues remark at my steadiness and presence as a signal that my mind and body are developing stabilizing capacities that enable me to operate with apparent ease despite my vision loss.

Awakening and Dissonance

Despite how hard I work, there are projects in which I am not so successful. Partly due to my progressive vision loss, but also due to my "learning curve," I sometimes fail to communicate clearly, manage my workload well, or understand what is expected of me.

In times of stress, I rely on the mistaken notion that if I just work harder, everything will work out. I stay later at night and retreat from lunch with colleagues, but soon become overwhelmed. I feel more and more isolated and wrestle to solve my work challenges alone. My desire to please others causes me to overcommit and make unrealistic assessments of what I can accomplish. I fall prey to the old adage that "a recipe for feeling overwhelmed is to always say yes and never say no." Sound familiar?

Then a partner asks me to step down from managing a new project because the partner and client are not satisfied with my performance. This comes as a big blow. I am devastated. This overworking, "pushing myself to my limits" strategy is not working. I feel like I'm an impostor and a failure. Now what?

Once the news soaks in and my emotional filters clear out the residue, I realize I need to take a break. I take a week off and attend a retreat at Unity Village in Missouri. I attend a Unity church in Washington, and the message "our thoughts are prayers" is seeping into my metaphysical pores. I have long wondered how to handle negative thoughts and fears, and the Unity message of affirmative prayer and gratitude seems to help me shift my thinking.

At the retreat, I feel buoyed in a vast reservoir of peace. I spend time in silence at the Unity Chapel and soak in the love. I attend a class on metaphysical or symbolic interpretation of the Bible, and the ideas and conversation reenergize me. With rest, loving support, and a change of scenery, my spirit revives. I sense that I am loved no matter what I do. Deep within, I recognize that all my striving may be getting in the way of a more authentic path—one in which I allow life to unfold.

With a renewed sense of clarity, I see that my life seems to be splintering. The roots of my spiritual life are drying up because of all the pressures and demands of my work life. I cannot seem to water both gardens at the same time without feeling an increasing dissonance in my soul.

So much of what is motivating me to work so hard is a subtle sense of shame. I compare myself to others who seem so self-assured. I counter these feelings by working harder. In meditation, I keep hearing the refrain, "You can never have enough of what you don't really want." When I'm busy chasing the external reward systems that surround me at work, I feel unsatisfied. My true longings for self-acceptance and connection with others seem remote. Once I am promoted to manager, emptiness and loneliness move in like a bad weather system.

As my vision deteriorates, I begin to make requests for accommodation. I speak to our project scheduler about specific work that will be difficult for me and work that I can comfortably do well. I produce a list of work activities that would be ideal given my vision. This move seems almost heretical given the strong work ethic in the firm.

I share with our project scheduler that I'm not well suited to lead in developing a proposal in response to a 500-page Request for Proposal (RFP) from a government agency because I have no way of motoring through that much material without any visual accommodation. I request a video magnifier like the one I have at home, but the human resources department doesn't take action.

The project scheduler says something along the lines of, "I'm sure there's something useful you can do around here." What a blow to hear those words. I have been recognized for several accomplishments, including winning a practice-wide award in past years. I imagine that her thoughts are reflective of the way others see me at the firm. I feel devastated and utterly powerless to do more work or do it differently. The jolt of being viewed so negatively pierces me to the core.

I seek coaching from colleagues in the firm as well as from friends with low vision. Inwardly I feel the tension between wanting to be successful and taking care of myself. I reach out to connect with a woman who is equally engaged in her career and also fostering her spiritual life.

We meet at my condo to talk openly about the challenges I face. At some point she delicately asks me what it is like for me with my vision loss. Her sincere interest, coupled with my fresh wounds at work, moves me to tears. She touches my grieving heart and all I can do is cry. All the busyness and striving fall away as I contact the emotions I have been pushing aside.

After our talk, I feel more whole somehow, more real. I experience a new compassion for myself. Over time, a clear and tireless ambition awakens within me. Perhaps this is about proving the scheduler wrong, or reclaiming my sense of dignity.

I refocus my work efforts and adapt to my challenges. I reinvent myself within the firm. I start with well-defined individual projects. I deepen my personal network of support. I begin taking better care of myself, exercising and eating well.

You might say I power through these times. I participate in large-scale projects and manage smaller ones. I facilitate a strategic planning process for a human resources department within a large government agency. We lead several groups through a "visioning" process based on a systems-level approach. This includes assessing and re-envisioning organizational components such as culture, leadership style, and systems.

We facilitate a session with lower-level government employees, including people in administrative and clerk jobs. This group also interfaces closely with agency employees serving as the HR "front line." When we ask the group to describe the ideal for each of these organizational elements, they can only speak about what is not working.

We listen and coach them to move toward the positive, but they do not. It's as if they can't dream about a different future until they process the tough stuff they're facing now. Eventually, the group is able to describe the ideal by flipping their current complaints into descriptions of what the opposite would look like. This teaches me to honor the emotional experience of loss and change with clients in the same way I'm learning to do so for myself.

Then I'm put in charge of a training development project with seasoned consultants from another practice within the firm. The role is fraught with clashing personalities and political dynamics beyond my understanding. I'm charged with overseeing the development of a new training program for one client while two senior consultants from another office are responsible for developing the material for the course. My attempts to support and enable the consultants to meet their deadlines clash with their needs to be in charge. The senior consultant managing the project allows me to take the heat without supporting me.

Ignoring the Costs

Up until this point I adapt to the hard edges of the work; late nights, last-minute travel, and the weighty tension of working within highly political environments all come with a cost. I can't see the impact because my "make it work" approach overshadows my sense of self.

I regularly pack Rolaids in anticipation of a particularly grueling meeting. When I have difficulty sleeping, I take a mild sleeping pill. The concierge at the Sheraton Manhattan seems more familiar to me than my friends and family. Job perks like riding in a limousine from LaGuardia Airport to downtown Manhattan and taste-testing from the room service menu lose their luster.

When I return from a week on-site with a client, I bark at the taxi driver who picks me up at the airport, full of mistrust and edginess by week's end. I find myself crying for no reason while at Nordstrom one day. By Sunday evenings I feel softened by time with friends and a chance to recharge. Tears stream down my cheeks as I pack my bag for the Monday morning flight. I ignore these signs for some time, until the light shines through. I realize that if I do not take some action, another year will slip by before I can exhale.

I realize I have made an unconscious deal with myself: hold onto this job so you're not forever on disability. I am doing it again—clinging to this job with the same fervor as my previous one. I care more about keeping the job than my own well-being.

One weekend while working out at the health club, I see someone fall while running on a treadmill. It is momentary chaos as this runner collapses and is ejected from the moving walkway. It dawns on me that I might stumble too—keeping up with the pace of my work life has become so automatic. What if I'm not on the right track? Slowing down seems hazardous to me. I need to find time to check in with my inner compass.

I enroll in a values-centered nine-month vocational program called "Working from the Heart." Program participants clarify their sense of purpose, gifts, and mission as a framework for creating the next chapter of their career life. I realize I want to work directly with individuals to support their personal and professional growth and well-being.

Slowly a spiritual change happens within me. I have what some have described as "divine discontent" in my work. I feel a subtle shift toward wanting to shape my career around a deeper sense of purpose, and feel the best way to do that is outside of my current role. I wonder, "Is this all there is?" I know I need time for discernment.

Creating the Conditions for Moving On

I see a counselor, and she encourages me to take stock of my experience at the firm. My work is beginning to affect my physical well-being. I still have no assistive technology at work, I'm fully engaged in my managerial role with several clients, and I keep hearing an inner voice nudging me to take time to consider my future.

I see the deepening values conflict within me. My desire to help and support others is at the core of my interest in consulting. The realities of large consulting work, the political dynamics, and even the work itself seems out of alignment with my growing sense of purpose.

We realize that if I am going to move on, I need to complete my experience there. As both a spiritual and emotional "truth and reconciliation" process, I honestly assess where I have contributed and where I have fallen short and what I might do differently. Over the course of the next year, I identify moments of pride, "broken promises," disappointments, and unexpressed gratitude. I meet with managers and one partner to acknowledge the above in our working relationship, and where possible make changes. I speak truthfully and respectfully to restore or establish trust in the relationship.

Gradually, one conversation and action at a time, I whittle away at my list. A passion for life emerges within me, as if I'm Ebenezer Scrooge on Christmas.[3] Withering resentments and self-righteousness are slowly replaced by self-respect and a newfound compassion.

The most daunting of these conversations looms before me. The manager who hired me is now a successful partner. Our professional paths rarely cross, and it seems so awkward to resurrect past difficulties between us. In conversations with my counselor, I search for the essence of my shortfalls while working with this manager.

For years, the stench of judgment and shame associated with this working relationship has kept me frozen in a straitjacket of self-blame. I feel completely responsible for the tensions and missed steps in our relationship. Many of his criticisms haunt me through my years at the firm, echoing long after our work is completed. I know I have to forgive myself before I can initiate a conversation with him, to relinquish the grasp of self-judgment and accept my struggles with compassion. Finally, I let myself off the hook for not being who he wanted me to be.

I schedule a meeting with him. As I approach his office, my throat tightens and I feel pangs of anxiety throughout my body. I enter his office, and we greet one another and sit at a small conference table across from his desk. After a round of small talk, I declare, "I wanted to meet with you to acknowledge my misgivings about my behavior in our work together years ago."

He leans back in his chair, crosses his arms, and replies, "I wondered why you wanted to meet with me, since we no longer work together. I suspected you wanted something from me." He shares his doubts about whether my proposed conversation is appropriate in the workplace.

I continue, "My interest is to acknowledge the ways in which I fell short in our work together. I am doing this for my own sense of integrity and don't want anything from you." I acknowledge the areas where I had regrets in terms of my behaviors and actions, and assure him that these are on my current radar screen. I do not make excuses or justify my actions.

He responds, "Yes, those are precisely the areas where I would have said you missed the mark." We talk a bit further as he reminds me that these same areas continue to derail me even today. I acknowledge the truth of his assessment. The conversation comes to a natural close soon thereafter.

As we approach the door of his office he says, "Now I do think that this conversation is appropriate in the workplace." I thank him and depart down the hallway to my office.

These tough conversations disentangle me from the past and enable me to leave the firm with integrity. They give me room to create something new in my career life. And that's what I do.

At a high point in my work cycle, I initiate conversation to go on long-term disability. It still feels as if I am leaping from a skyscraper window, without seeing the net below me. Even with tremendous inner clarity about my need to press the pause button on my work life, I consider ways to be on disability part-time and still work with select clients. Letting go of my role altogether seems such a daunting step to take. Thankfully, I am discouraged from setting this idea into motion.

I clean out my office. While I don't know what's next, I feel I am saying "yes" to something inside me.

Seeing Our Wholeness

Ultimately our journey is toward wholeness, which requires letting go of outdated roles, thoughts, and behaviors to come closer to who we are meant to be. Life has a way of nudging us in that direction by putting obstacles in our path that force us to grow. This is at the heart of transitions:

letting go of the old to embrace what we can't yet know we will become. When we are ready to move on, we find a way to do so. This requires a willingness to plunge into the chaos of the unknown.

It takes courage to move into a transition and be willing, like the snake, to shed the layers which have come to define us in order to move on. For those with a disability or life-altering challenge, moving on when it feels right is even harder.

Simply dealing with the unwanted physical challenges or changes can all too easily become our primary focus in life. So to take a risk to honor our wholeness, knowing it may be difficult, takes tremendous courage. As we trust in our wholeness, we let go of the handrails that roles and identity afford us and approach that which naturally enlivens us. This process of transition includes a reawakening of energy and momentum as we voyage through uncertainty to a new and distant shore. Ultimately we emerge renewed, changed, and reawakened in the process.

Take a moment to look back on your life. When have you had to let go of an identity, a role, or a way of being? Where has that letting go led you and how has it increased your wholeness? And what are the thoughts that keep you from embracing that wholeness in its fullness?

A coaching client started her own art business while working full-time in an office job to move toward more fulfilling work. A mother of two returned to graduate school to start a new career built on her life's passion. Each in her own way moved toward positive change without knowing how things would work out. Initiating positive change takes courage, and facing illness or life-altering loss only makes this more complex. Seeing our wholeness reminds us to consider what we want, what is best for us, and what step will enliven us.

The first step in seeing our wholeness is uncovering where we are not seeing ourselves fully. Journaling, working with a therapist or a coach, or conversing with trusted friends reveals distortions in our sense of self. Rather than blaming others for not valuing and respecting me, I had to learn to value myself.

I was doing what I call "pretzling" myself—twisting myself out of shape to get the work done, hiding my visual challenge, ignoring the costs to my well-being—and it took some reflection to recognize that I was blind to my wholeness. People might not have valued me as I'd have liked, but the real power for me to change was inside me.

The clues were all there. All the times that I felt wronged, victimized, and treated unfairly were indicator lights. As I unpacked each situation, I could dismantle the self I had come to see and consider new possibilities. This practice of deconstructing how we see ourselves is both daunting and liberating. I suggest good company when exploring these outmoded beliefs, since to this point we have not been able to dismantle them alone.

As we face choices in our lives, we begin to orient around our wholeness. We may still listen to our fears and doubts, but we start making decisions from our strengths based on what is true for us when we are at our best. Ask yourself, "What do I truly want?" When we do this, we affirm our wholeness. Turning down job offers builds our sense of integrity when fear would be our sole motivation to say yes.

Honor yourself in your decisions. Consider what transitions you might initiate if you saw yourself on a journey toward recognizing your wholeness. Don't allow the vulnerability you may feel because of your difference or challenge to squash your impulse to move toward your dreams.

Be inspired by my legally blind friend who left her work staring at a computer screen all day to become a health and wellness coach. She connected with her passion and gifts by cooking, coaching, and publishing a cookbook.

Consider your well-being as integral in the choices you face. Begin to bring all of yourself into decisions you make and to steer yourself toward greater well-being. See the many ways you contribute, positively influence others, and thrive. Begin to contemplate your value apart from anything you do or accomplish. Shine the light on areas where you are tolerating behavior or situations that drain or diminish your life energy.

If you're holding back from being yourself at work because you think you are somehow "not enough," think again. If you choose to come out of hiding about being differently-abled, which is the fabric of your life, you reveal your humanity and sense of self. You accept your gifts as being enough and don't have to constantly prove you're okay. Like me, you stop rejecting yourself because of this difference.

QUESTIONS

What does it feel like when you see your wholeness? In what parts of your life is this happening?

PRACTICE

> When you encounter situations in which you do not feel whole, journal to discover and deconstruct underlying self-perceptions that are no longer useful to you. Engage a positive and supportive friend, coach, or therapist in conversation about what you learn.

CHAPTER 3

ACCESSING DIGNITY

"If you limit your choices only to what seems possible or reasonable, you disconnect yourself from what you truly want, and all that is left is a compromise."

—Robert Fritz

Moving into a whole new set of daily rhythms excites me. For so long my work obligations defined my priorities. Being able to design my own schedule thrills me. I feel a sense of creative energy arise as I imagine all that I can do with this time. Who knows what my life will look like?

The very week my leave begins, I fly to California to participate in a weeklong clinic to learn alternative medical therapies to improve my sight. Grace Halloran, the workshop leader, has explored various healing modalities for her own sight loss from retinitis pigmentosa (RP).[1] The course is attended by folks with various chronic eye diseases, mostly RP and macular degeneration.

I don't know why I've been so open to alternative healing approaches, except that ever since I heard my eye disease was incurable, my competitive spirit wanted to move beyond this life sentence. Someone I met offered a different interpretation of incurable, suggesting that it really meant that the allopathic medical community had not yet discovered a cure.

Grace trains our class on a regimen of acupressure, the use of a TENS[2] unit around the eye acupressure points, color light therapy, and a Touch for Health[3] protocol. After the first full day of therapy I walk out of the Bay Area hotel and am immediately struck by how yellow the taxis are. In fact, all colors are more vivid. It's as if I'm watching an old black-and-white movie that has been colorized. A flood of hope streams through me

Throughout the week, our learning community works together, helping one another and laughing at times. Grace verbalizes almost everything for the benefit of those with little sight. I find this comforting. I immerse myself in the healing regime, and vow to keep it up once I'm home. I purchase a TENS unit and continue all the daily therapies.

These therapies result in improvement in my vision. The treatment does not reverse my eye disease, but the improvements are remarkable nonetheless. Months later, I schedule an appointment at the National Eye Institute, a part of the National Institutes of Health in Bethesda, Maryland. Every few years I spend a full day there as a part of their ongoing research protocol. The tests capture the progression and state of my disease in great detail. Results include a graphic depiction of the scotoma or blind spot within each eye. Other tests measure color vision and acuity.

As part of this process, the doctor asks me to read the eye chart. Once I do so, he looks puzzled. He scratches his head and folds his arms, as if something isn't right. He says he wants to measure the distance between my chair and the chart. He retrieves measuring tape and verifies that the distance between the chair and the chart is correct. I read the chart again. He doesn't understand how my vision could have improved. I explain that I have been doing several alternative therapies for months. I don't think he actually registers what I am saying.

I think I am helping medical science by performing my own clinical trial and am now offering the wonderful news to him. But he doesn't see it that way. He finally pronounces that I have experienced a "not insignificant" vision improvement. I hand him a research paper documenting results of the use of the TENS unit on patients with macular degeneration. He seems to disregard most of what I say, and I suspect he will not read the report.

One of the lessons I learned from this experience is that we see what we expect to see. The doctor had trouble seeing the vision improvement, in part because his years of clinical work and research solidified his expectations. I didn't fit into his experience with the multitudes of patients he had studied. This experience reminded me to track my openness to healing and possibility and to watch how tightly I hold on to my narrative of vision loss.

Once I began to see myself as whole regardless of my "disability," I took hold of the direction of my life. By being true to myself, I gained access to dignity and integrity. That's what I wish for you.

In this chapter we will unpack the power of dignity. Dignity is defined as inherent nobility and worth; being worthy of honor and respect.[4] In my journey with vision loss as I became "differently-abled," I struggled anew with issues of worth and value. I discovered and slowly relinquished my accumulated negative beliefs about illness and my sense of worth.

Self-respect is at the core of accessing dignity. Without this foundation, we cannot operate on our own behalf in the world. Connecting with my inherent goodness helped me to act with dignity and respect for myself. Taking a proactive stand for ourselves and how we manage our time reinforces self-respect.

The Tyranny of Freedom

Upon my return from California, I begin to piece together a daily rhythm. No more commuting, client meetings, and squeezing errands in between my "real work." I have so many choices. I face a new challenge—how should I structure my time?

At first I orient myself around caring for my physical well-being. I start attending a weekly regimen of yoga classes at the nearby health club. I trade in my business suits for yoga clothes. I spend time cooking healthy food, folding in nutritious leafy green vegetables in accordance with Grace's suggestion.

But I am 39, and relatively healthy. I may have a disability, but I still want a full life. I have time on my hands. Staring at the empty calendar is daunting. It's as if I switched trains halfway through my trip; the slow steam-engine pace feels foreign after riding the bullet train for so many years. While at the firm I fantasized about having time to really take good care of myself, but now having virtually no constraints feels uncomfortable. I recall days spent home from school in childhood and the awkward feeling that I was missing something and was somehow left out of "real life." Questions of meaning and purpose percolate up. What am I going to do with my life now?

Thus begins another life and career planning cycle for me. I liken these times of exploration to discovering the many branches of a growing tree. In the search for the "ideal mix" of career, volunteer, social, personal, and spiritual dimensions of my time and life, I need to listen deeply and experiment. This enables me to create my next life chapter.

When I first explore a new branch, I don't know whether it will be a side trip or the continuation of the core foundation for my future. Either way, I can learn from the exploration, because I'm gaining clarity about what really matters to me.

Months later I am contacted by the founders of Working from the Heart about becoming a part of their leadership team. Founder Jackie McMakin has dedicated years to helping others find meaningful work and is ready to move on.

She contacts recent alumni who have expressed an interest in supporting the organization's work—it's time to hand the work over to new leaders. A group of coaches, trainers, and passionate alumni form a working group. We develop a series of train-the-trainer materials and workshops to capture and transfer the learning acquired by the founders over the years.

I am grateful for the chance to use my gifts with a group I so value. I plunge into visioning and planning meetings, sub-group work designing the train-the-trainer sessions, and meetings with Jackie. The rich interchange I had so enjoyed while consulting is revived as I work with dedicated and inspiring people on these projects.

Ultimately I decide not to pursue a leadership role within the organization. The possibility for financial sustainability is just not there, and I also feel hesitant to take on someone else's baby. I want the opportunity to design new material rather than work with materials and designs which are already finely polished.

Meanwhile, low-vision aids proliferate, which make my life easier. I start working with screen magnification software that enlarges and reads aloud whatever appears on the computer screen. I also discover optical character recognition (OCR) software, which revolutionizes the way I read books. By placing an open book flat onto a scanner, I scan the book and the software recognizes the text, displays it on the computer monitor, and reads the pages out loud to me. This means I can read whatever I want independently. I no longer have to limit my reading to what is already available in one format or another, or request that a volunteer read aloud or record a book for me.

Life Beyond Work

I also participate in other values-based career and life-planning seminars. In a three-day LifeLaunch workshop I examine my life direction.[5] As I stand back and look at what is becoming more important as I am approaching my 40s, a lightbulb goes off in my head: what about life beyond work? One of my peers in the LifeLaunch workshop develops a mission statement that really gets my attention. Her goal is to "love and be loved," which makes me realize how much a significant relationship is missing in my life.

The stimulating professional relationships I've developed, coupled with the long hours and travel, contributed to my fulfillment in work. I've also developed close friendships with several women who were traveling similar professional paths. I certainly have dated, and have the battle wounds to prove it. But my work demanded so much of my time and energy that I'd neglected the personal side of my life. This is one of those times when myopia blinded me to the bigger picture.

Am I too late in the dating game to settle in with someone special? Do I possess the skills to navigate such unfamiliar and seemingly treacherous waters? How much will I need to learn to be successful in a committed intimate partnership? I'm afraid I may not even be capable of such a relationship. I wonder whether my vision challenge will be a nonstarter for prospective dating partners. First dates are designed to screen out prospective partners based on the proverbial "checklist," right? This is why accessing my own nobility and self-respect is so important to me as I enter this arena.

I slowly begin to flirt with the dating world. One of my immediate lessons is that time spent in other relationship arenas is no substitute for the emotional intensity and anxieties that are unique to dating. When on first dates, I center myself while paying attention to my internal experiences.

Afterwards, I go over my residual impressions for clues about next steps. Years ago a visually impaired friend shared feelings of disappointment about not having a family. She said she was so preoccupied with keeping her job that she never pursued marriage or family. I don't want my vision loss to stand in the way of finding partnership.

Tangled Up All Over Again

Within six months of going on disability, I've created a dizzying web of commitments and responsibilities. Between my commitments with Working from the Heart, pro bono consulting for nonprofits, and a burgeoning social life, I'm overwhelmed.

Interestingly, the patterns that plagued me at my previous job have traveled with me to this new life. Why does this surprise me? Because even though I believe and have experience with my personal power to create and make things happen, some sliver of me still blames life's challenges on outside forces like employers.

The facility with which I have re-created the same dynamics proves that I am the creator of these situations and serves as a motivator to change my inner patterns. For example, I question my belief that I need to operate from a place of constant overwhelm. Maybe I can create spaciousness in my daily routine and give myself room to breathe.

Meanwhile, all the purpose-oriented exploration I've been doing has opened the door to a new chapter in my career—coaching individuals in transitions. I attend coaching training offered through Newfield Network and the Hudson Institute. I start working with people I know who are interested in making a career transition.

During the Newfield training, I receive wonderful coaching. I talk with my coach about setting reasonable expectations in my work and personal life.

I begin to work with new patterns in these arenas of my life. I learn how to design conversations and agreements that build trust. In my personal relationships, I practice making clear offers and requests. This is new. I've been more comfortable sulking when my unexpressed expectations were not met.

I also learn how to design conversations without collapsing into my emotional vulnerabilities. A new vision of communication emerges in which I can stay both open and connected during an exchange, granting another person space to decline a request or making a counteroffer that stems from my wants and needs. I am amazed at how much easier relationships are when I take the risk to make clear requests in a place of equanimity, which allows the other person to share in forging an agreement that is workable for both of us.

I date a man for several months who seems to have all the right stuff. But I feel unsatisfied, wishing for more. From the start I sense he doesn't regard me as especially significant in his world. Between his job, his child, his other commitments, I feel squeezed in—or perhaps squeezed out.

At this point my coach invites me to be proactive in shaping the relationship through making clear requests. I feel "one down" in the relationship, a scenario in which it is nearly impossible to make requests, particularly bold ones. The same "one-down" orientation that accompanied me in my work is showing up again. Seeing myself as less attractive because of my vision subtly skews my thinking and actions.

My coach keeps reminding me that my brewing dissatisfaction is worth paying attention to. It points to areas where my needs and expectations are bubbling to the surface and wanting attention. I make respectful requests to my male friend regarding my concerns. His responsiveness affirms my trust and hope in our relationship. Eventually, I make a request that creates our breakup. Although I feel disappointed, I gain a sense of dignity and power, knowing I have shown up fully and boldly.

For me, it is also about practicing saying no. As requests for pro bono consulting come my way, I discern inwardly whether or not it is a fit, and then often say no. This new move enables me to navigate from my own sense of priorities and resist the impulsive temptation to please others. I experiment with how to best support others in practicing these principles in their lives.

I receive a call from a colleague at my old firm. He wants me to consider coming back to serve in a newly created role. The company is developing an infrastructure to support employees in career planning and work-life balance. Somehow it all seems too good to be true. It's an ideal job description, given my passion for career coaching and my experiences learning about balance and work-life issues.

Something in me is clearly resisting this opportunity, however. My emerging intuitive voice sends signals of hesitation and doubt. I honor this impulse and decline the opportunity. Months later the colleague tells me that the firm decided not to staff the proposed department.

Trusting My Experiences

Slowly my anxieties lessen and a sense of trust about life emerges. I can't say at exactly what point this happens, but I've traveled to a new place of acceptance, not just tolerance, of my continual vision loss. Things are actually much more "okay" than I imagined, and I'm beginning to feel my hands on the steering wheel of my life.

In addition, leaving the consulting firm with dignity prepared me to accept just how much power I actually have to manage my own life. I have become comfortable using technology that makes reading and working on the computer very workable. Through the use of one technology or another, my thirst for learning can be quenched.

Although I miss the many stimulating connections with colleagues, I form several professional and personal relationships. With two other colleagues we create a "visioning group" to birth our emergent career paths. We meet monthly to explore our individual possibilities.

Through all of these activities, it is such a relief to honor the rhythms and natural patterns that support my well-being. Maybe I can find new and unchanging ground in being present for my experiences and deepening my relationship with myself. This awareness of a new way of orienting represents a different way to move through life.

Occasionally I catch glimpses of an emerging spiritual perspective. A question such as "What am I meant to learn here?" comes to my mind. When I experience serenity I value the peace I feel. I contrast this with my habitual focus on external circumstances. It's as if I am looking down from a mountaintop, and with the horizon before me, am able to put things in perspective.

I affiliate with a group of "new age" thinkers, exploring metaphysical writing such as the Course in Miracles. The course focuses on spiritual sight. With frequent references to "seeing differently" and forgiveness, the course asserts that healing occurs when we "see" through a lens of wholeness rather than as separate selves. Fear creates perceptions that drive us to protect ourselves from others. The question from this way of thinking that continues to hold long-term interest for me is, "How can I create more peace by seeing this differently?"

Perhaps my vision loss was pointing me toward my greatest life learning, to a question that I didn't altogether consciously choose, but one I was living in: "How do I see myself, my life, my world?" My vision loss made this question a rather obvious one, perhaps, but it was one that had haunted me for a long time. Throughout my life, I've been naturally drawn to spiritual texts that focus on seeing differently, healing the way we see, and forgiveness.

Living in Three Worlds

More and more I notice I am living in three distinct worlds. One is made up of people who understand the experience of vision loss and adjustment. It includes low-vision support group friends, specialists in the field of low vision, as well as nonprofit leaders and advocates dedicated to improving the world for folks experiencing vision loss. In this world, there are also people I meet with whom I share a quest to conquer long-term health or life challenges and thrive.

Then there are people who may or may not know about my visual loss, but with whom I disclose only what is necessary to coordinate some transaction. Ticket agents at the airport whose assistance I request to print my ticket and servers at fast food restaurants whose help I need when ordering fall in this category. Also included here are friends whose curiosity to understand my experience does not intersect with my comfort level in disclosing details of my daily challenges.

There are others who do not know of my vision challenge, given that it is not readily observable, or with whom I don't disclose much about my experience. This includes strangers and acquaintances and others who have no clue about my visual challenge.

In all these worlds, I don't want to be defined solely by my physical challenge. I start to pay attention to what it is like to disclose my visual difficulties to others, seeking ways to retain my sense of dignity. I begin to understand the differences between being differently-abled, being independent, and possessing dignity. Self-respect and dignity are not contingent on being fully-abled or healthy, as I once unconsciously presumed.

I explore ways to ground my sense of self beyond my limitations so that I participate more fully in conversations. I soon discover that I feel better when I take responsibility for creating an energetic and bodily sense of strength while in these conversations. Any hint of wanting to be okay or be liked throws me off balance. The fact that I am compelled at times to disclose my visual challenge in order to interact with someone can resurrect feelings of insecurity. If we find ourselves wondering if some aspect of our identity will adversely affect the way we are treated, we may be experiencing oppression.

I do not want to be swept into another's negative rendering of vision loss or health challenges. Because of my early experiences hiding my vision challenge from students, I start each training session with a disclosure. But I don't want the focus of our collective attention to be on my "disability."

Through this investigation, I realize I value the sense of ease I feel in the world of those who understand what my experience is like. I don't have to explain myself or educate them. I also see that I have to articulate my needs and requests in the other world so that people will begin to understand my needs.

My greatest learning about diversity, including the experience of being "out" or "one down," comes to me through being legally blind. Not only is the world set up for fully-sighted people, but society trends toward a baseline of normalcy around sight. Handouts at meetings, name tags, elevator buttons, and signs all assume 20/20 vision. So the onus is on me or anyone outside the norm to explicitly request some form of assistance or accommodation to access shared information. Anytime others respectfully join me in getting these needs met, I feel less alone.

I've read that as we change emotionally and spiritually, we may find that we need to update others on who we are becoming. We translate ourselves anew in long-standing relationships. We do this by showing up in our new and evolved way of being, and hope we can find common ground with the folks we have known for a long time.

During this phase of my process, the intention that is taking root within me is to access the dignity within. One way I can measure this is by how fully I am living and thriving despite my vision loss. Early in my journey, my identity was fused with my visual challenge, and I saw myself in terms of what I could no longer do.

As I begin to see my wholeness, dignity also resurfaces. The dignity inherent in my humanity enables me to advocate for my own well-being and make choices based on what I truly want and need. This dignity stems from turning toward my experience, accepting and loving myself.

My vision loss profoundly shapes my life, and my actions and reactions are inextricably linked to the experience of having 20/20 vision and then gradually losing it. I'm tethered to this unavoidable stone in my path. But as I learn to see through a new lens, I continue to find meaning—and dignity.

Accessing Our Dignity

As I chronicle my experience of this gradual yet occasionally frightening loss, you can recall your own experiences when things didn't go as you'd hoped they would and how you navigated through these times. Perhaps you'll recognize yourself in my letting go and moving on from difficult and unanticipated challenges. Whatever your loss, I want you to join me in discovering the resilience of your soul and spirit to reclaim your dignity. In Japanese, the word for resilience translates as "struggling well." Recall the strengths and gifts that enlarge your life during tough times.

We begin by seeing what is possible, but not yet manifested. Where are we so closed to possibilities that our life collapses into itself? Is fear painting such a vivid picture that we no longer see clearly? Somewhere within we access an opening that tells us it may not be so bad, even if we cannot know this for certain. Dignity enables us to imagine again.

We may stop granting complete authority to experts to define our future. We claim our power to dream, to imagine what might be possible, even beyond our circumstances. We dare to take time to listen to what we want as a way of honoring ourselves.

We find our own rhythm and model our lives around that. We access the power of exploring options and then saying yes or no based on what enhances our life energy. Ask, "What else?" and "What is missing?" when it comes to creating a vibrant life. We move from survival to possibilities, and then choose from those options.

Dignity is not defined by circumstances but by how we live. There's dignity in pursuing our dreams and honoring what inspires us. A blind colleague reminds me that when he coaches others and offers mobility training, he distinguishes between asking for assistance and retaining the right to direct one's life.

Needing help or support does not mean we are delegating our path and choices to another. We can make requests and offer to do what we want to do more of. We can say no when it's right for us, even if it makes us squirm. We stop trying so hard and trust that by showing up and doing our best, we are doing enough. We listen for a life-defining question that propels our learning.

Questions

What inquiry is calling you to live fully right now? What is a vision for your life that completely energizes you? What would thriving look like for you here?

What structures and support do you need to thrive?

Practice

Declare your intentions when you face a challenge. Decide how you want to be in the situation, what living fully and from your sense of dignity would look like here. Commit to this with a friend.

CHAPTER 4

ORIENTING FROM PURPOSE

"I think that most of us are looking for a calling, not a job. Most of us, like the assembly line worker, have jobs that are too small for our spirit. Jobs are not big enough for people."
—Nora Watson, interviewed by Studs Terkel in *Working*

The "neutral zone" of my career transition from management consulting to the independent life was characterized by a deep desire to land. I longed for a place and time where life would settle into predictable patterns and rituals. Being supported by long-term disability relieved me of the pressure to perform. This enabled me to pay closer attention to aligning my work with my true sense of passion and fulfillment.

In this chapter we will explore meaning, passion, and fulfillment linked to work and contribution. Your challenge may have indeed led to a job loss or perhaps the inability to work for a living at all. If it hasn't, I invite you not to wait for a break such as being on disability to listen to your inner longings for fulfilling work. No matter how differently-abled you are, honoring your calling crystallizes momentum and fulfillment.

We'll explore some of the traps that prevent you from honoring your true calling and see how to listen for clarity. You'll begin to identify the essential ingredients for your best work. Intentionally addressing these questions equips you to live fully. Lining up your work with your inner sense of meaning and fulfillment is like tuning yourself to your soul, while ignoring impulses to seek greater alignment detracts from your aliveness and sense of dignity.

As I work on raising my standards for living in alignment with my sense of purpose and passion, I increase the meaning and fulfillment I experience. For me, thriving means trusting that the best ways to express my gifts will become clear if I genuinely seek greater alignment.

While at the consulting firm, I explored my sense of purpose by asking what truly mattered to me. I rediscovered my deep concern for how people engaged while at work. My vision for healthy collaboration and respectful communication emerged and brought new focus and momentum to my consulting work.

Toward an Inner Compass

As I continue to search for the best use of my gifts, time, and energy, I think that if I can just figure out what I am called to do, to know my true sense of purpose in life, then I can relax. I don't recognize the myth behind this notion. I've read just enough books like *Do What You Love, the Money Will Follow* to be consumed with finding just the "right" path for me and the false belief that it is an easy thing to do.[1] Finding the perfect work gets promoted to my life's elixir. Sound familiar?

My sincere desire to align my work with my soul becomes an obsession. In the terms of Christian scripture, it becomes a false idol. This is not the first time in my life that a heartfelt urge has taken on larger-than-life dimensions. For me, it is a little like starting down a country road and ending up on a superhighway in under a mile. Underneath the quest for my ideal work there lies a lot of anxiety. I hitch myself to the star called "find right livelihood" and think if I only can follow that star, all will be well. I have more work to do on myself.

At work in the past, I often misplaced my needs for fulfillment and validation by seeking them from those who were critical of me. Challenging personalities and low-level office politics distracted me at times. I felt unable to move or shift from being affected by these dynamics to navigating from my sense of personal power.

I was drawn to consulting largely because I valued helping others. Over time, I took on the firm's clear reward systems to the point that my sense of motivation became obscured. Every month we managers received reports which ranked us in two ways. One ranked us from highest to lowest year-to-date billability. The other ranked our year-to-date sales.

I'm not naive enough to think that a consulting firm could remain in business if it did not track these two performance measures. Yet paying more attention to such measures than to my spirit created tension and internal conflict.

Now I yearn not only to return to the active workforce, but also for work to be in greater alignment with my values and well-being. Taking that next job will mean losing my disability benefits, so there is an incentive for me to make sure the fit is very good. I consider the disability benefit a safety net to support me in a transition to my next job. My unknowns include how much of a workload I can sustain using my new assistive technology, and how closely the work can mirror my emerging sense of purpose, passion, and aliveness.

Taking time to deliberate about what matters most to me, I realize that I have a deep desire to help others discover their sense of meaning. My in-process but working purpose statement becomes "My purpose is to help others articulate and live fully into their sense of purpose."

This conscious awareness impels me to set clear intentions and organize my actions around what I care about. A greater life energy emerges. Psychologists call it flow. How I get to this point is the result of a series of experiences.

Learning to Listen

One summer, I go on a retreat in Massachusetts. The retreat house is operated by an Episcopal order of brothers who reside in Cambridge. Unlike other retreats I've attended, this individual retreat lacks formal group participation, structure, and leadership.

Apart from occasional meetings with a spiritual director, retreat participants direct their own time and experiences built around shared silent meals and services. Each participant stays in a hermitage equipped with bedroom furniture, a meditation bench, a writing desk, and bathroom.

I have some concern that since I have not carefully selected a workshop with just the right theme, I may not get the spiritual support I need. I wonder where the substance will come from without a retreat leader or guide.

My first full day there, I indulge in as much outdoor activity as is humanly possible. I canoe in the pond, hike along the hills to a beautiful overlook, and explore the property. It's as if I've signed up for Outward Bound instead of a silent retreat.

By the end of the day, I have accumulated so many mosquito bites that my legs actually hurt. I count 45 bites in all. All the attendees have their own way of settling into silence, and my way seems to be by wearing myself out.

I find myself returning to a wooden bench at the top of an overlook, where I can gaze at the vista below. I spend quite some time perched there, just sitting. My spiritual director suggests that what I am doing parallels my life stage. I am at a place where I want to gain perspective as I look over my life. I gravitate to that spot because it affords me the ideal setting for this reflection.

By the end of the week it becomes clear that while there was no agenda, retreat leader, or structure, I got exactly what I needed. I feel spiritually met and tended to by some greater wisdom. There's a familiar saying about retreats like this. You come thinking it is about this or that, and leave knowing it was about something altogether different.

Listening more actively becomes my staple when reading, writing, and learning. I am an interactive learner, so comprehending through listening takes work. I often close my eyes while listening to books on tape, both to sharpen my concentration and my imagination. When editing a document on the computer, I close my eyes and listen for patches of dissonance.

Listening inwardly becomes another arena for expanding my awareness. "What is the quality of this inner prompting?" I ask, and then, "Is there a sense of spaciousness or is that ambivalence?" "Does this thought enliven my energy or soothe my spirit?"

Distinguishing flatness or dull sensations from enlivening ones becomes useful when I'm making decisions about next steps. If I experience a sense of dullness in my heart and chest area when considering an action, I wait till a thought produces an energizing sensation in my body. Often I sense excitement as streaming or pulsating energy around my abdominal area that suggests aliveness. I allow the sensations in my body to inform me, and I allow this information to guide me. This represents a whole new way of orienting for me, a different way of "seeing."

Listening for a New Career Direction

In the spring of 2000 I take a big leap. I enter a process to consider becoming an Episcopal priest. This is a specific process run by the church to evaluate a person's potential and capacity to be a priest. Raised as a very inactive Unitarian, and exposed to a Christian youth organization for high school students called Young Life and the Baptist church in Indiana where I grew up, I experienced a slow but certain conversion process. Or maybe I would call it a spiritual awakening.

As long as I can remember, I sensed there was some power greater than myself. As a young girl I often felt held and supported when I walked alone in nature. I recall being atop a mountain in Colorado at Frontier Ranch Young Life Camp and feeling a sense of God, or Jesus, being with me.

As a teenager, my way of testing God one night was to ask him to stop my hiccups while falling asleep. The hiccups abruptly stopped after my silly little prayer. I was "saved" one Sunday evening at the nearby Baptist church as I felt responsive to the call from the minister to step forward to the altar. In all of this, I brought a genuine desire to connect with a larger sense of spirit.

However, I became disenchanted while at the Baptist church when people who claimed to have been saved were privately smoking and drinking and flirting at church camp. My young spirituality was fragile and affected by hypocrisy as I watched those around me in religious contexts. My shallow faith was easily overshadowed by other high school priorities, such as being included in the popular clubs and events, trying out for cheerleading, and shopping for clothes at the mall. In my 20s as I began to face physical and emotional challenges that intellect alone could not resolve, I began seeking spiritual sustenance through meditation, prayer, reading, and conversation with others.

Feeling resistant to Christianity, given my exposure to hypocrisy in church, I was more open to Eastern religions and spiritual practices. I began experimenting with prayer and meditation and finding out what was truly useful for me. My pursuits were linked to relieving my suffering, overcoming the negative self-talk, and the challenges I faced.

I wasn't interested in intellectual exercises around belief or dogma; I wanted a spiritual life to guide me in living wisely. Serenity and peace were among my top priorities. In true seeker fashion, I explored various communities of faith, spiritual retreats and workshops, and held many rich conversations with fellow inquirers. Somehow I was also wanting to "land"—to have a home base for shared spiritual life and learning.

At the suggestion of a good friend, I attend an Episcopal church in downtown Washington. Almost immediately I feel engaged. The sermons are not only relevant, they also help me in my day-to-day living. A friend invites me to enroll in a four-year program entitled Education for Ministry (EFM). This program, sponsored by the University of the South, parallels seminary training, but requires less commitment of time and money. I say yes without fully thinking it through because it seems like an answer to my prayers.

A small group of us meet on Monday nights at the church to discuss our weekly reading. We apply a theological reflection process to a particular issue or situation in order to explore spiritual perspectives. Once we share our "spiritual autobiographies" with one another, it becomes clear our religious upbringings and beliefs vary widely. I find the scholarly reading and commentary to be accessible and credible.

The conversations in EFM are rich, and I'm developing the kind of fellowship I never experienced in a religious community before. As a single woman with a demanding career living in the city, it offers me a family setting, for which I have long hungered.

Taking Exploratory Steps

I become active in the church, facilitating half- and full-day retreats on topics such as applying spiritual principles in the work setting. I find a natural intersection between spiritual principles and the soft-skills training I've been doing with leaders around interpersonal communications. Bridging these worlds and facilitating conversations with others awakens my sense of vocation and passion.

I receive training offered by the Christian Vocation Project and the Listening Hearts Ministries. The focus of this work is to facilitate others in living their sense of purpose and call. As an expression of faith, how might God be calling one to act in the world? The invitation is to encourage one's faith and spiritua life to inform one's work in the world. This doesn't mean everyone should be a minister in the church setting, but that a God-centered inquiry around work, meaning, and contribution can provide direction and clarity.

I'm asked to serve on the committee to help a fellow parishioner discern her possible call to ordained ministry. To discern is to distinguish meaning among the many voices within. The committee work follows a clearly outlined process of inquiry and discernment.

One of my personal outcomes of this effort is a yearning to express my growing spiritual foundation more fully. I feel as if I've compartmentalized my growing reliance and trust in God, or perhaps set it aside at work. I am not interested in evangelizing, but I'm so energized by spiritually focused conversation.

I take these questions to a spiritual director whom I met during the Working from the Heart program. My central question at this time is whether to stay in my current work or to move on.

My spiritual director asks what the quality of my thoughts and feelings are when I think about staying in my current role. She asks, "Is it like a drop of water hitting a rock and running down, or more like that of a sponge, soaking in the water?" I suppose the sponge conveys emotions and states of ease, abundance, and calm. I'm clear that not all spiritually centered decisions feel this way, but there is a rightness that the sponge metaphor offers me. Regardless of the seeming difficulty of the path or choice, is there more of a sense of love or peace in one choice than in another?

Discernment as Spiritual Decision-Making

Discerning what God, or my inner wisdom, is calling me to do is different from making decisions. The word "decide" comes from the Latin *decidere,* to cut off. To decide is to cut off or to kill options, similar to suicide, homicide, etc. Feeling a need to decide evokes a quality of control and managing. Metaphorically, it conjures up a sense of reducing or eliminating, even making some options wrong at the expense of others.

Discernment, on the other hand, involves listening for a sense of clarity to emerge. This is an active process. To listen for the subtle distinctions and nuances of internal yearnings and impulses requires patience. Discernment includes recognizing patterns and trends. According to the book *Listening Hearts: Discerning Call in Community*, certain signs indicate that a call comes from God:

- Peace
- Joy
- A temporary experience of disorientation, followed by calm and serenity
- Tears that are comforting and tranquilizing, rather than disturbing and fatiguing
- A sudden sense of clarity
- Strands of experience that seemed unrelated begin to converge and fit together
- Persistence: the message keeps recurring through different channels.[2]

As I'm discerning my next career steps, I notice a trend in my spiritual life. A subtle inner prompting to "give back" begins sounding in me. When I witness examples of others acting out their faith, I notice my quickening attention and a hint of envy. There is an opening up of possibility that these examples create within me. An inner excitement coupled with a cognitive recognition—such as, "Oh, work could be like this!"—arises in me.

Discernment in Community

When I enter into the discernment process for ordination in the Episcopal Church, I have to consult a variety of people. I meet with the bishop, my peers from around the diocese who are also considering priesthood, and a committee that forms to support the process within my church. Regular meetings with the priest at my church punctuate the process, and meetings with other clergy also shed light on my discernment. I feel both excited and daunted by stepping into a public role in my faith life. Until this point, I shared my faith with those with similar mindsets in a peer-to-peer type of mutual disclosure.

Still, insecurities about how the church would view my vision loss linger. At an employment conference for visually impaired job seekers, I listen to a poignant story of resilience told by a panelist. This totally blind woman in her 20s recounts her trials interviewing for over 50 jobs. After each rejection, she wonders if showing up for the interview with a guide dog diminishes her chances for a position. Her buoyant spirit effervesces throughout the audience as her positive attitude and message touch us all. She eventually lands a job as a procurement specialist with a government agency.

For a low-vision conference, I lead a session entitled "Follow Your Career Passion." I speak candidly with participants about time on disability leave from work. I share tools I used to clarify my sense of purpose, gifts, and passion. Participants engage fully in the exercises.

The deep determination and resilience I witness in their examples inspire me. They too wrestle with vision loss taking center stage in their careers. Moving from "What can I do?" to "What do I love doing?" seems like a luxury given that the majority of those with vision loss do not return to work after going on disability.

Steps Toward Healing Vision Loss and Work

I meet an Episcopal priest who has experienced vision loss. We talk on the phone and meet when she visits Washington. Here is someone who has similar sight challenges, and yet she is among the first women to be ordained in the church. She served as a parish priest and also taught at a seminary.

Her commitment and humility inspire me. She shares how she is able to read from the pulpit and perform other priestly functions. What a gift to meet someone who has already overcome one of my own major stumbling blocks to priesthood. Her experiences clarify both the challenges and workarounds of being a priest with vision loss.

The rector at my church encourages me to become a reader for Sunday services. He suggests that the congregation needs to see me perform in that critical function. Based on what I learned from others, I prepare the scripture reading on a set of PowerPoint slides using a large font setting. I rehearse at home for the Sunday reading until I feel confident.

When Sunday arrives, I carry the PowerPoint deck to church. I feel my palms sweat as my time to read approaches. A sense of self-consciousness, of being uncomfortably thrust into the center of the stage, swells within me. I ask myself why I have taken on this crazy challenge as a legally blind person. What am I thinking?

As I read in front of the congregation, the anxieties dissipate. I have grown to love the passage I am reading, and somehow hearing my own voice and these lovely words take on a life that overshadows my concerns. As I return to my seat, I catch the smile of a friend who has made the pilgrimage to my church just to witness me reading.

Through the discernment process, my faith and gifts move to the foreground and my "disability" label moves to the side. In the parish setting, the workshops I facilitate touch people to approach work in a spiritual way. Once again, as my sense of purpose lines up with the work I am doing, my dignity arises. According to theologian Frederick Buechner, vocation is where our gifts and talents meet the world's greatest needs.[3]

Instead of thinking about decision-making as only an intellectual and reflective process, try discernment. It invites experience and experimentation. The analogy of a sailboat with the sails out and the rudder guiding below, as it glides through the water, conjures up images of learning through action. Taking steps toward a particular direction will allow for experiences that crystallize where you are being called to serve. That's what happened to me.

Way Closes, Way Opens

Despite my sense of calling, anxiety stands out most prominently among the emotional qualities I experience during the formal ordination discernment process. There is an absence of joy, peace, and calm. The joy which is so palpable when sharing with fellow seekers seems missing. It's as if the petals of my spirit have all but disappeared, like a rose in full bloom turned toward winter.

In addition, early in the process, my priest confides that he has received a call from a fellow parishioner offering her vote of "no confidence" for my future as a priest. Other people express tension and dissatisfaction with the church's discernment process. The whole thing doesn't feel right.

When I finally meet with the bishop to hear her decision regarding my future in the church, I am ready for the process to end. Her decision that I should not go forward to ordination produces feelings both of deep rejection and of relief. What part has my vision loss played in the decision? Or are my Unitarian roots and meditation practice simply too far out in left field? Am I too unconventional or unsophisticated to be a priest?

The bishop wonders aloud if my current work, consulting to organizations, training, and coaching, is in fact my true calling. She invites me into the inner sanctum of consultants working within the diocese as a way to integrate my spiritual life and work. Ironically, a few years later, I become quite engaged as a consultant to the subsequent bishop, leading strategic planning and facilitating leadership retreats.

As with most other job searches, the bishop, the ultimate employer, makes the final decision. It seems natural to focus on this outcome—I wasn't chosen—and overlook my lessons during the process. What am I learning about which contexts enable me to thrive? When am I most alive and engaged? Paying attention to what we still have to learn is hard to do when we have been rejected. Yet as the Quaker Parker Palmer says, "Way closing" can be as informative in discerning God's call as "way opening."

As is often the case, I come to see that the process unfolds with much grace. I realize that my burgeoning spirituality is not linked to a specific profession as a priest. However, I don't need to disavow the growing role of spirituality in my life. One of my greatest lessons of this time is that I am being called to be more open about my spirituality.

Some force is calling me to live outside the bureaucracy and career structures of church life. Once I am willing to relinquish my tight hold on a defined career grid within which to plot myself, I become open to further honoring my internal wisdom. Apparently I am being called to travel even further out to sea, to invent a career and a life outside the norm, and this calling is the best way to cultivate my trust in an inner knowing.

Looking back, I see that I had to let go of the formalized roles and structured institutions that might well have strangled my spirit and aliveness, because God or some force greater than me saw promise in my capacity to not only work through the unknown and unseen but to lead others through this territory.

The fact that the universe did not allow me to settle into a defined career track necessitated an even deeper spiritual life for me. It's as if attaching myself to a clear career path inside a hierarchical organization was a temptation to abdicate my internal compass. The temptation was thwarted, and I had to return to deepen my own spiritual well.

Recognizing a Calling

The change in direction leads me, at the encouragement of my parish priest, to develop an eight-week program for parishioners entitled "Discerning Your Call." I witness fellow parishioners' sincere desire to align their sense of spirit with their work or volunteer efforts. I sense their deep passion as they recall times of doing their best work. I also feel the pain of disenchantment and loss of dignity with careers gone sour. I wonder how anyone with a spiritual life could answer questions of vocation and purpose without dipping into their spiritual well.

Sometimes our greatest moves are a series of small steps—so small we hardly notice them. I facilitate the discernment series twice at my church, and participants share their experiences with others. A few participants ask me to provide some follow-up coaching to support them individually. A parishioner asks if I will be her job coach.

Suddenly people begin to come to me for support during career discernment and transitions, and particularly want to view their progress in a spiritual context. In a way, it's the perfect intersection of my passion and gifts. I have survived two major career transitions, received training as a coach, and am seeking ways to express my values around spirit and work.

Unhitched from my prescriptive instincts to put myself in a defined career box, I begin to allow my inner sense of energy and aliveness to guide me in my career choices. My vision loss serves as a prompt in my own path to heal my career. By accepting the constraints created by my vision loss, I allow my innate strengths to shape my career path.

What I see now is that over the years, there was a gradual alignment within me, as I slowly began to do my best work without attachment to what that should look like. Joy and aliveness became the clear indicators pointing me to my most naturally fulfilling work.

Truing Yourself to Your Values

You probably hear echoes of your own life in my story—your desire for a meaningful life, as well as the accompanying challenges and obstacles that you must navigate. What I'm hoping is that you also get a sense that by turning inward and moving through these challenges from a deep inner core, you'll find your way to your heart's desire.

In my work with others as well as in my own life, I witness over and over again the power that comes from the fundamental shift from anchoring one's life around an employer or a job to orienting around an inner compass. As we recognize themes in our best work experiences, we become comfortable with the idea of enjoying work and honoring our passion, and as doors close as well as open, we redefine the basis for making choices about our work.

Here is how this exploration often unfolds: When the tension of feeling "out of sorts" grows to a certain point, clients contact me to explore ways to realign their sense of values in their work. I witness their innate desire to have integrity in their work and relationships.

They will say things like, "I know I'll be taking a pay cut in this transition, but I'll feel better about the work." Underneath this statement, I hear a resounding need to recapture dignity, to realign their work life to mirror their prized values. Often a client's exploration of meaning and purpose coupled with reducing stressors will renew life at work.

Studies have shown that the number-one reason people leave their jobs is because of the dynamics with a boss or other colleagues.[4] I help these folks navigate through these interpersonal waters to access their sense of power and authenticity.

At the beginning they talk about being snagged in challenges and problems they don't sincerely care about. The surrounding culture dominates their field of concerns until they are swept into the system's quagmire of conflict. I ask, "Why is this concern important to you?" Or, "How much energy and attention do you want to dedicate to this concern?"

Discerning which challenges or problems to focus on enables clients to manage their energy. There are always unsolvable problems in our midst, and they offer ripe temptations which divert us from our deeper sense of purpose. We cannot ignore the impact of office politics, yet we can make choices about how we manage our energy, emotions, and attention.

Many of my clients experience what Frederic Hudson described as the "doldrums."[5] They have lost their sense of passion and energy for their work. Yet they hesitate to make a move because they really want greater fulfillment. Leaping to the next job and hoping it reinvigorates them does not feel like the right approach anymore. A change of scenery alone does not solve the problem. They want to be sure the next move is right for them.

As the sands in the hourglass of our lives diminish, our desire to live fully quickens. We may be more impatient with the ways we have put up with circumstances. We may also feel more responsibility for ensuring our sense of fulfillment and meaning.

Those experiencing chronic health challenges often face an intensified yearning for meaning and fulfillment. A visually impaired friend is an example of tireless dedication to improve the quality of life for those with vision loss. After leaving a consulting firm, she returned to graduate school. She leads a local nonprofit, serves on community boards, advocates for disability-related issues, and embodies a genuine sense of joy.

When I start working with someone who is in the doldrums, they usually speak with fervor and clarity about what they do not like about their job, their boss, the culture of their organization, etc. It seems impossible for them to stay focused on what they want.

In our work together, as they reconnect with their sense of purpose, the gifts they most want to use, and their power, they begin exploring possibilities oriented around the "sweet spot" of their best work. Reflecting on their highlights in both career and other areas of life enables clients to identify the essential ingredients for fulfilling work.

Joanne was a senior-level attorney within a government agency who experienced the same kind of divine discontent I had when consulting. An Ivy League grad, she worked tirelessly for years to ensure justice and equality as she rose within her federal agency. She served as an acting senior executive, yet felt ambivalent about whether to apply for the job itself.

When Joanne hired me as her job coach, she took a step toward shaping the next chapter of her career life. She is successful, well paid, and has attained a high-level position in her field. But she is unhappy. Stifled by the politics and bureaucracy in her work, she has lost the passion that once inspired her. Her work life is stale and draining. She is worn down, like the dull edge of a once sharp knife.

What unfolds in our work together is a reawakening of her spirit and energy as she faces her work stressors and covers new career terrain. How does she do this? She envisions work more in alignment with her personal sense of purpose and those gifts she most wants to use.

We begin our work with an activity in which Joanne identifies several memorable high points in her work and life. She writes about what made each experience engaging and fulfilling. We discover the key themes and map these to the gifts she most wants to use. She recognizes that her current work is lacking these essential ingredients, and considers the possibility of redefining her work around these gifts and interests.

She eventually liberates herself from that which drains her and takes a leap to a career that affirms her passion and inner compass. She takes a leadership role in a nonprofit. She enrolls in seminary and volunteers within the church. Her sense of joy and aliveness surges.

Embodying Purpose

In 2003, I attend a retreat for people with chronic illness. The weekend retreat is held at a nearby convent center. It's the result of efforts by a woman who has been diagnosed with multiple sclerosis (MS). The retreat planner demonstrates such nobility. When asked about her participation, she says, "I want to attend tomorrow's session, but I will not know until I wake up if I am able to do so."

She stands out as a living example of what it is to accept and not be defined by one's limitations. She projects a sense of humility about how her disease confounds her, but a peace that tells me it doesn't define her. I suspect her faith creates a container that is bigger than the MS in all its challenges. To me, her very presence communicates a sense of equanimity and purpose. Her gifts of wisdom and peace touch me. She reminds me that how we live can often demonstrate purpose better than what we say.

I witness many who get caught in the grief cycle and don't possess this kind of acceptance. She must have encountered sore points in her process of loss. It seems to me that there is dignity in befriending whatever experiences arise around a trauma or chronic illness. Perhaps it is more "being with" our fluctuating emotions while not getting swallowed by them that enables the kind of dignity and humility I encountered in the retreat leader.

This retreat recasts chronic illness as an opening to a deeper union with God. Those of us facing continual loss may choose to enter these places alone or with others, including a force greater than ourselves. For me, it was the only way I could navigate through the loss and disorientation I experienced, never expecting fruits such as a more God-centered life or a deeper sense of intuition to follow. I do see now that one's purpose may be to "wake up," as the Buddhist would say, or to live a "Christ-centered life," as the Christian might say.

I once saw a black-and-white film clip of Viktor Frankl speaking to an audience of death-row inmates. He described the opportunity in any moment, even our last, to define meaning in our life. He said even loving one other person creates meaning and purpose. His experiences in a World War II concentration camp clarified for him the power each of us has to define meaning for our lives.

Accepting What Is, Embracing What Is to Be

It's no surprise that acceptance, in the Elisabeth Kübler-Ross grief process, comes after so many stages of emotions. I know for me a sense of peace and ease arises when I finally accept "what is." Yet this seems unimaginable when I'm at the beginning of a loss or transition. Many of us get glimpses of acceptance along the way, however. I experience these as a "settling into" the realities of a situation, without a focus on what's next, or even what could have been. There's a quality of not grasping, or needing things to be different.

In transitions, there comes a point when we accept our current situation. We see that some of our hopes have not been realized and others have. We imagine that although we might have done some things differently, we are ready to move on. We are propelled by some combination of wanting to move on and aspiring to some new direction. Our longing to seek greater alignment with our sense of purpose moves us to take some action.

Musician and author Robert Fritz, in his book *Path of Least Resistance,* highlights the "creative tension" that arises with awareness of our current reality and vision for the future.[3] Our experience of this creative tension is part of what propels us toward our vision.

He gives the example of a person who goes on a diet and wants to lose 20 pounds. When the weight gap is at the greatest point, the dieter is motivated to be successful. Somewhere after the midpoint, however, many dieters lose steam and motivation. The tension lessens as the dieter approaches her goal weight.

Fritz suggests that we harness this tension to become a creative force in our life. Without a vision, most of us tend toward the path of least resistance, which seeks the lowest point, like the water running down the mountain stream. We naturally orient around our problems and challenges. If we aren't careful, at the end of the day we end up resolving difficulties, but we fail to focus our energy on creating new frontiers. By claiming a future, we focus this tension and orient around what matters most to us.

We face enough obstacles, distractions, and challenges in everyday life to occupy all of our attention and energy. Whether it is interruptions or politics at the workplace, or just staying ahead of one's obligations and the logistics of living, we can have the experience of swimming upstream just to stay where we are in life. Under stress, many of us orient even more around those concerns that most challenge us, preventing potential difficulties. But it doesn't have to be that way.

Questions

> Some say a true calling is the work you must do, either because you are filled with a strong passion to make something happen or because of your unique set of life experiences and perspective.
>
> If you could only dedicate yourself to one goal or mission, what would you do to further this in the world? If you knew you could not fail, what would you do next? If you had the opportunity to broadcast one message to the world, what would your message be?
>
> According to Martha Finney, co-author with Deborah Dasch of *Find Your Calling, Love Your Life,* "There are only three real reasons why we are paid to do anything: to bring beauty, to relieve suffering, to restore hope. That's it. Whether you pack carrots for a living or are a neurosurgeon. It all comes down to one or more of those three things."[7] Which reason most resonates with you?

Listening for Purpose and Vision

When you find yourself in a transition and don't know what's next, listen for a sense of "what wants to happen." Recognize this as an active process.

I've even developed visions during difficult personal losses. After ending a relationship, I developed a vision for how I wanted to move forward. First I identified my top fears and concerns. I was primarily worried that I would become bitter and disenchanted as I moved into dating. I set an intention to be open-hearted toward myself and others. This conscious intention helped me to focus, particularly when grief arose.

Gradually listening for what wants to take shape in your life gives way to vision. Pick up the new threads born from genuine longing, as if the seed, finally rooted, sprouts, and the life force propels you forward to bear new fruit.

I started working with a mid-career professional who was experiencing stagnation and a sense of the doldrums in his work. We explored his prior peak experiences, which revealed his love of problem solving, research, and analysis.

I asked him to develop an ideal job description based on these elements. Every time he sat down to craft the description, he came up blank. Finally, I asked him to draft a description of the job from hell. He developed this within days. Then I asked him to draft a job from heaven by flipping the negatives into positives. Once this was complete, the picture became concrete—even possible.

His enthusiasm about the work he really enjoyed motivated him to find roles that actually excited him. After exploring several options, he decided to accept a promotion within his department.

Orienting Around Purpose

I invite you to move squarely into the questions "What would enliven me even more fully?" and "When I'm thriving, what are the essential ingredients of my best work?" Let your body and emotions answer these questions even more than your thinking mind.

Taking steps to explore options adds to the inner reflection about your direction. Pay attention to the trends and patterns in your life. As you read the tea leaves of your desires, take steps to explore what truly enlivens you. Let the momentum that comes from doing your best work reshape the canvas of your work life.

Practice

Your path might look something like this:

- Notice and explore dissonance while working/contributing.
- Follow your internal desire for greater alignment.
- Reflect on your highlights and identify the essential ingredients of your best work.
- Weave more essential ingredients into everyday activities.
- Create a vision for your ideal work.
- Make specific requests of peers, employees, or managers to enrich your fulfillment in work.
- Take steps to move toward your vision.

Question

What would living into your sense of purpose more fully right now look like?

Practice

Pay attention to your aliveness and energy as you contribute.

CHAPTER 5

Cultivating Embodied Wisdom

"Within my body are all the sacred places in the world, and the most profound pilgrimage I can ever make is within my own body."

—Saraha

As you read in the last chapter, my clarity around purpose produced a greater alignment with my gifts and values. Yet I still longed for an inner navigational system for living. Could I intentionally cultivate the greater wisdom of my mind and body as I navigated through life?

When coaching, I experience a great sense of energy and notice a similar liveliness in my clients as they zero in on their purpose and passion. It's this rise in energy which is a key indicator that a person is on his or her path. Now that I notice that sensation in myself and others, I wonder what else my mind and body will reveal if I just listen. And I wonder what I could help clients discover in themselves if they could tune in to their embodied wisdom more.

That's what this fifth strategy is about—how to connect to and cultivate a rich source of inner guidance so that you can live ever more intentionally, no matter what your circumstances. So many of us live from the "neck up"—disregarding important signals and being driven by others.

By cultivating a relationship with my body, I gain access to greater wisdom and presence. My vision loss disoriented me in both practical and emotional ways. It intensified my already finely tuned orientation toward pleasing others. By working with somatic practices that calm my mind, I create an inner stability which is observable to others.

Steadying ourselves through the body enables us to have more ease and calm. For those with a disability or illness, calming the mind and body can really enhance clarity and focus. By proactively building our capacity to withstand the stressors and tensions in everyday life, we develop resilience.

Learning Through the Body

In 2005 I further my coach training through embodied leadership study with Richard Strozzi-Heckler at the Strozzi Institute in Petaluma, California. Richard is trained as a psychotherapist and an aikido practitioner, and he studied for years with Dr. Randolph Stone. Dr. Stone developed Polarity Therapy, a healing modality which seeks to restore balance and release blockages in the energy systems within the body. Richard and Dr. Robert Hall developed a form of bodywork which releases the armoring one develops in response to life's challenges, thus affecting the self through the body.

The Strozzi Ranch is situated in the hills outside of Petaluma. The arid landscape is enveloped by the large azure sky. The pastures are speckled with horses grazing amid the quiet. Classes are held at the dojo, which translates as "place of learning." Aikido practices form one of the foundations of the somatic work.

Small groups form to meet and witness each member "tell their professional story." Telling our stories authentically and persuasively offers a chance to get immediate feedback from our small group on the impact of our message.

Capturing highlights of my "professional autobiography" evokes a sense of pride. I feel a sense of amazement as I track the learning and evolution of my work and contribution over the years. I marvel at how many supposedly "missed turns" yielded fruit over time.

As I enter into this course of study, I experience a wave of deep sadness, tied to adjusting to many life changes, including vision loss. Due to a professional commitment I arrive on the second day of the training. In catch-up mode, I lunge into a small group activity, offering my story to a team of relative strangers.

Richard strolls in and sits right next to me as I'm preparing to launch into my "authentic marketing pitch." I feel thrust uncomfortably into the limelight; grief hovers right under my skin. My throat is tight and waves of anxiety roll through my musculature. This is not how I want to feel just before a presentation.

At the end of my "telling," Richard speaks with depth and clarity, "There is nothing about the way you move that conveys you have limited sight. There is a way that your experiences of vision loss have shaped you, and made you a unique coach and consultant. What has developed in you through these experiences?"

My throat tightens. I reply, "I just try hard." I feel the tears slowly making their way down my cheeks. Waves of grief stream through me as I recognize the impossibility of this worn-out approach in my life.

He invites me to refrain from trying hard for the duration of the course and to pay attention to what emerges instead. Trusting the wisdom of my body, I could resist acting on my pusher-driver instincts. But hasn't my body already disappointed me with vision loss and now food sensitivities? How can I trust my innate bodily wisdom?

I will have to let go of believing my body has betrayed me. Gradually I become curious about how my body is artfully adapting to the vision loss despite my conditioned tendency to move into overdrive. This is the perfect assignment for me. Doing less, not more, is a new strategy.

Finding Ground

The training offers a number of new ways of being. For instance, I've often heard the phrase "finding my ground," and now I have a chance to explore what it means for me personally. Phrases like "to thine own self be true" come to mind. I'm a person with real physical constraints—I don't know what the future holds for healing. I am independent, yet I rely on others at times for support.

Richard challenges us to stand on our own two feet and center. Centering is the process of being in the center of our mind, body, and spirit. In language, silence is the center. It can be a place of openness, of space for listening and for inspiration. In our emotions, acceptance is our place of center. In the body, one is centered when still and when accessing our physical center: that point just below the belly button and in the middle of our body. And for our spirit, center seems to be peace, equanimity, and perhaps the breath.

As I stand, I allow my center of gravity to take shape. With the full support of my legs, my back, and my feet contacting the floor, I arrive in the moment.

Generating a bodily sense of stability and ground by centering myself affords me a felt sense that I can savor. A felt sense refers to a set of sensations in the body that are distinctly experienced and recognized. I want to live this way. I want to build the trust in my own body so that I can be guided by the impulse to move that comes from my belly, not from my head. Perhaps I can track my internal cues for movement, for action, for speaking, and even for inaction. When does my body say "no" or "not this way"? What are the cues that translate into "no"? And conversely, what are the signals and sensations that indicate "yes"?

Misty of Chincoteague was a book about a fabled wild pony who was bought at the annual auction held to pare down the size of the wild herd.[1] The ponies are rounded up once a year and led across a narrow strait from Chincoteague to Assateague Island, Virginia, where they are auctioned off. The herders also provide veterinary attention to the ponies that make the trip.

In order to provide the safest passage for the ponies, officials time the swim to occur when there is neither a low nor high tide. That way the water in the strait is not rushing in or out quickly due to the tides. This temporary calm in the waters ensures safe passage for the ponies.

In the minutes between the tides, the ponies travel from the shore of one island to the shore of the other island. The joke that is often told is that if a TV film crew pauses while the network goes to commercial, they risk missing out on live coverage of the whole swim.

This is a great metaphor for centering. Those times of internal stillness enable us to pay attention to our inner life. These quiet places often go unnoticed. At times I need to create these safe, still moments through silence and meditation, as the saltwater cowboys did for the wild ponies.

When I center myself using somatic practices such as focusing on my belly and relaxing my whole body, I experiment with placing my thoughts on the back burner. Allowing the wisdom within to express itself without intervention enables me to honor the quiet voice inside.

Creating a Sense of Embodiment

What does a sense of embodiment mean? Most of us focus on the activity in our mind. We track our thinking, or consider our world from the perspective that our mind reigns as our master or guide. When I began meditating regularly, I recognized that my mind was subject to habitual patterns of worry, scrutinizing the past and trying to work out the future.

Although a tremendous resource, my mind regularly got stuck in these patterns. This "hamster mind" runs on its exercise wheel as part of its conditioning to protect and preserve. A state of mindfulness occurs when we are aware but not attached to what is happening in our mind and body. The more mindful I am, the more I see these thought patterns as mental habits rather than "the truth." When I anchor my thinking in my body by becoming fully centered, my thinking shifts. Thoughts seem to arise from a deeper well altogether—perhaps my own intuitive wisdom.

Practice

Try this centering practice for yourself. Allow five minutes and sit or stand in a quiet space. With eyes open, but not actively looking at anything in particular, take at least three deep breaths, inhaling so that your belly expands. Be sure to exhale as long as you inhale, even longer if you can.

Be determined to become centered. Feel your feet as they contact the floor or your shoes. Pay attention to your physical body, concentrating on sensations such as pulsing, streaming, and even areas of numbness. Feel each sensation from the inside out. Relax your shoulders and any other part of your body that is tense.

Become aware of the full length of your body. Imagine roots extending down below your feet like those of a tall tree. Feel the full length of your body and beyond. Imagine a core stream of energy running from 10 to 15 feet below your feet, continuing up through your spine and extending another 10–15 feet above your head. Inhabit this sense of length, bringing your attention to the felt sense within your body. This dimension of center represents dignity.

Now, focus on the area surrounding your body. Imagine spheres of energy surrounding you. This second dimension represents width. Fully occupy the space around you, as if it is your only task. You may imagine that each time you exhale you are expanding your width further and further. This is the domain of relationships and community. Consider fully inhabting your own width and at the same time connecting with others around you.

Finally, locate a point within your body, three finger widths below your belly button and at the center of your physical body. Locate your thinking and even your breathing in this place. If you get distracted by thoughts, simply return to the focus on your belly center. This is the dimension of depth, where you access what matters to you.

Notice and take in the sensations you are experiencing. You can do this practice anytime—either on a regular basis throughout your day or just before an event that might be a trigger for your nervous system. Notice what parts of your body relax when centering. This will give you clues about where you hold tension.

Over time, centering and other somatic grounding work creates a core deep within me. I relinquish extraneous concerns and dedicate myself to the work that fully enlivens me. The uncertainties I face externally about my sight are steadied by my growing sense of center.

I begin to orient around what I really care about, including listening for the truth of my experience. Until now, circumstances and others' opinions dominated my worldview. I ignored my own thoughts and sensations about my experience.

Later in the program year, we explore intuitive and sensate awareness. We stand face to face with our eyes closed and sense into each other. The exercise pushes the boundaries of my understanding of sensing others.

Richard announces in front of the class that when it comes to this work, I am like an exposed raw nerve ending. The words pierce through me like a sword. The teacher whom I so admire is calling attention to one of my vulnerabilities. I feel a heaviness, a surge of tears, a swelling of my throat.

As soon as we break, I gallop out into the fields for a long-awaited private cry. I ask myself, "How come I am so sensitive? Will this ever change?" At this moment I can only see the price I'm paying for my sensing capabilities.

As I stand hugging the fence outside, tears streaming down my cheeks, co-trainer Susie Nichols gently approaches me. I explain my hurt and humiliation. Somehow in all of this I took Richard's comment as a criticism. My patterned response to such rejection is immediate escape. It doesn't occur to me that he is affirming my gifts.

Susie encourages me to explore the meaning of Richard's assessment and mine it for its true value. I realize I digested his comment whole, without first chewing on it a bit and tasting its richness. The next day I ask Richard for clarification, and am able to take in the affirmation of my intuitive capacity.

We talk about ways to manage energetic boundaries, something I didn't even know was possible. How can I explore this intuitive capacity further? I've always wondered how much of my struggles have been shaped by being so open to others. Is negative energy contagious to someone like me? What can I do to manage my energetic core? Could deepening my intuition help me navigate in the world of deteriorating physical sight?

Can you relate to this attitude toward your sensitivities? Are there areas of your life that seem more like vulnerabilities than strengths? Can you imagine how these same aspects are also gifts both to you and those around you?

Just as we identify gifts that seem more like vulnerabilities, we also work to build strength in our body. We practice embodying resilience as we notice ways our bodies shut down in the face of challenge. We are asked to focus on a goal that we imagine to be situated at one end of the training room. Two fellow class participants stand facing us at the midpoint with hands held up at shoulder height, creating a human blockade. We are told to move toward our goal and to notice what happens as we approach this human barrier.

The first few times I approach my classmates, I slow down. I feel uneasy pushing past their outstretched arms, even though I know they have been instructed not to lock hands so as to prohibit my passage. I lose sight of the goal altogether. It takes several rounds for me to reengage with the commitment to my future that is just beyond the blockade. This remains a powerful reminder of how quickly I orient around what is getting in the way and how deeply invigorating it is every time I rededicate myself to the vision that energizes me.

The more I practice centering and other embodiment practices, the more I choose new responses, the more I take conscious charge of who I am becoming, no matter what is happening to me.

Accessing center is crucial in finding ground, especially when the ground I have known has shifted. For those experiencing illness, centering yourself enables you to trust and relax. If, like me, you have lost trust in your body, feeling as if it's not on your side, centering unveils places of steadiness and calm. Experiencing this inner strength can restore your trust in yourself. Silent retreats, somatic centering practices, meditation, and contemplation all have heightened my felt sense of center.

I often begin a coaching session with the centering practice described above. Then I ask clients to speak from the "physical center of their body, just below the belly button." This point happens to be where a number of major energy meridians intersect according to traditional Chinese medicine. It is also the place from which aikido practitioners anchor and move while on the mat.

Learning About Intuition

I become deeply curious about embodied knowing and intuitive sensing and want to explore it further. A coaching colleague suggests I contact Desda Zuckerman. Desda founded CoreIndividuation, an energetic healing modality.[2] While on one of my trips to Petaluma, I meet with Desda and experience her work. Afterwards, I feel lighter and more embodied.

I find myself talking with Desda about her upcoming four-year CoreIndividuation Apprentice Training Program, all the while not sure how I've come to consider it. I don't see myself becoming a healer. The body of work is complex. I've done so much professional development in the past years and I'm not sure I want to do more right now. My interest centers on deepening my intuitive and somatic awareness to compensate for my vision loss. I want to "see" as clearly as possible in whatever ways I can.

I tell Desda that my real aim in becoming an apprentice is to deepen my inner sight. She applauds my quest. She tells me she expects her apprentices to become CoreIndividuation practitioners after four years of study. Despite my ambivalence, in 2007 I start.

Decades of Loss and Adjustment

By this point in my life, I've experienced decades of vision loss. I'd gone from enlisting volunteers to record books to using computer software that reads to me. In my early 50s my acuity approached 20/400. After two bike-car accidents, I stopped riding my bike. I started riding tandem bikes with a friend when at the beach.

I could no longer read my own handwritten notes, even though I used a large black felt-tip pen. I began taking my small laptop to conferences and workshops to take notes. I gave my first PowerPoint presentation in 20 years using the dual monitor function of my screen magnification software. This enabled me to project a regular-sized font onto the screen while viewing enlarged letters on my laptop.

I placed large print letters on the computer keyboard, along with bump dots on certain keys, to use as markers for my hands when typing. I placed bright yellow bump dots on my kitchen appliances—the oven, microwave, and toaster oven—to mark temperature and on-off settings.

I bought my first smartphone with a built-in screen reader and began texting friends. I started attending audio-described opera performances and actually understanding the subtitles and what was happening on stage. I purchased a talking scale which, when prompted, will say hello, share my current weight with me, and say good-bye. Now I call a local number and can listen to over 100 newspapers and magazines from around the country read by a computerized voice (NFB Newsline).[3]

As I write this, I am struck by just how much loss, experimentation, and adaptation has taken place during these years. I'm fond of so many of my low-vision aids, yet I recognize that this was not always so. I don't think there is one low-vision aid that I wanted to use until I really needed it. I much preferred doing things the way I had always done them, the way everyone else did things.

And the unexpected pleasures also surprised me. Listening to books on tape reminds me of childhood times spent listening to my mother read to me. I cuddle up on the couch, perhaps with a blanket if chilly, close my eyes, and dial into another world. Every time I weigh food or myself, the talking scales voice a pleasant "good-bye" when done. I can't help but smile when I hear this.

These experiences of vision loss also called forth responses from my body. My ability to hear, to listen deeply, to empathize and to be guided from within emerged with the loss. Who knows if I would have heard my inner voice so keenly without vision loss?

But once listening becomes a pathway for learning, I want to call upon this resource more fully. Some part of me is still seeking wholeness, which includes filling in the gaps left by my sight loss. Without realizing it, I was also seeking deep healing.

Listening to the Body for Wisdom

In the fall of 2007, I attend the first of many training sessions as a CoreIndividuation apprentice. Our class is made up of coaches and healers trained in nursing, homeopathic medicine, acupuncture, craniosacral[4] and massage therapy. We are drawn to the CoreIndividuation work and dedicated to healing ourselves and one another in this laboratory of learning. Looking back on this time, the deep healing and the intimate mix of dynamics, it is difficult to put into words the myriad of experiences and emotions.

CoreIndividuation is healing that supports the authentic and full expression of the energy which includes and surrounds our physical body. CoreIndividuation is ancient work and cutting edge at the same time. It draws on wisdom from many healing arts, such as acupuncture and energetic work taught by Dr. Gayle Pierce. But it builds on these, using discoveries by Desda Zuckerman after 45 years of research

This healing work addresses and impacts the emotional, spiritual, physical, and mental aspects of our well-being. It is grounded in a state of embodiment and engages the client in partnership. The work is noninvasive and profound at the same time.

The CoreIndividuation practitioner facilitates a move toward wholeness by clearing debris, supporting realignment, and releasing blockages in partnership with the client.

I witness transformation in my own life and with others. Most often, there are periods of great intensity just before an apprentice training is about to get underway. Since we participate as both healers and clients, we perform healing work on one another as we learn the work. We also work with a number of apprenticeship clients throughout the program.

During this time, another challenge is weighing on me. CoreIndividuation practitioners refer to several three-inch binders while working with a client. These volumes include graphical depictions of the energy anatomy, descriptions of over one hundred procedures, references to maps, and details of the structure and healing protocols.

In order for me to read print materials with any degree of confidence, they need to be at least 28-point font. How am I going to amass the material into a form that I can easily access? I'll need to pull a wagon behind me just to carry large print versions of all this material when meeting a client!

At a low-vision technology trade show, I learn about a machine used by blind and visually impaired individuals to listen to books, podcasts, notes, and other media. I ask the salesperson if it is possible to download text files onto the handheld Victor Reader Stream machine.[5] Yes, as long as I convert the files to Notepad, I can organize, bookmark, and recall select pages relatively easily. I purchase the Victor Stream, which my classmates and I call "Vicki," and access most of the information this way. I create one volume of graphics and a large print index of all the procedures for my reference during healings.

A New Identity

Up until this point I haven't seen myself as a "healer." My identity as a management consultant and business professional overshadows this possibility. I know I won't be a healer who appears through a doorway of hanging beads wearing a flowing, multicolored new age gown. But then again, nobody in our class fits that description.

In 2009, Desda holds a ceremony in which we each receive the "healer's mantle." During this ritual, she speaks our virtues as individual healers. We all have been developing our own ways of sensing and seeing. I receive an invitation to "see" with a multitude of "eyes" and to trust what is coming to me.

I am inspired to "see" the healer within me and expand my horizons. And I begin to see how all the dark places I've inhabited have prepared me to support clients as they faced similar challenges. As with coaching, my experiences of loss and gradual transformation enable me to bring a sincere empathy and hope to others in their journey.

Desda challenges me to stop seeing myself as visually impaired. Here is someone with heightened intuitive sight challenging my narrow interpretation of sight. She illuminates the many ways she has witnessed my sight expanding over the course of the apprenticeship. Intuition, inner sight, imagination, inner listening, vision, and deep empathy were all ways she has sensed my sight.

Paying Attention to the Gifts

While I don't believe God or the universe caused my vision loss, I'm very clear that it's brought focus to my life. I'm one of those people who get lost in possibilities at times; my mind just seems to keep generating ideas and options.

With greater difficulty in reading, I must make more choices about what to read. When a certain activity becomes challenging, I ask myself if it is worth it. This compression of possibilities or narrowing of options serves to focus my life. This is a big help to someone like me. New constraints provide the challenge and focal point for innovation.

Although some activities are simply off the table, I've deliberately continued those I deeply value. Perhaps this is where dignity lives. If I opt out of an activity for my safety, I retain my dignity.

Painting is one of those activities I indulge in, even though it is wearing on my neck and back. Since painting is a relatively new pastime for me, I don't get caught in the swirl of regret, wishing it would be "like it used to be."

One of my fellow low-vision friends demonstrates the value of focus. He is a father of two and manager within a government agency. His vision loss started in his pre-teens, and advanced rapidly. He describes his role as referee for his kid's soccer team. It's the only way he can be engaged with them as they play. He gets right into the action and tracks what is happening. He uses every bit of his limited sight to stay engaged with his kids.

Physical challenges may only appear to be concrete barriers. The human spirit is fierce, creative, and committed to a greater realization of life than we might imagine. To some, the physical challenge is part of the creative tension, with a compelling vision providing the fuel for stretching beyond the expected.

Changing Somatic Conditioning

Our bodies, like our minds, are capable of change. Even though we think of our bodies as solid and defined, we are able to shift and change our musculature, which informs who we are as humans.

I'm not talking about working out at the health club. I'm talking about such things as melting away bands of armoring around the chest and heart area, for example, so that our shoulders are not caving in (as mine once did). The narrative associated with caved-in shoulders might include a defeated wearing away of confidence, for example.

Thoughtful coaching and physical practices can support the release of this engrained story and the body that holds it. My listening and observing as a coach deepens as I begin to track my clients' subtle distinctions in the body.

One client holds her head facing downward as she describes her work. Her gaze tilts toward the floor with a mood of disenchantment at her sense of being stuck. As we shift this story and the way she holds herself, she enters into new territory. The body changes to reflect inner changes. She looks directly at me as her face lights up. Her chest softens and her gestures portray excitement as life energy emerges. Her conditioned tendency to orient around her work and live from a mood of discouragement proved strong but not fixed.

In my work with a newly promoted senior government manager, we discuss her lack of confidence when in senior staff meetings. Over the phone, she details her somatic "caving in" as she becomes so critical of herself during meetings that she rarely speaks up. She zeroes in on feeling "not enough" and comparing herself to more experienced managers. At these times her body feels tight as her chest contracts due to shallow breathing.

I introduce her to centering practices over the phone and notice her voice markedly soften and deepen. She becomes calm and deliberate as her breathing expands into the belly, and she reports that her shoulders and jaw relax. She takes this practice into senior staff meetings and reports she is able to experience this same sense of calm. She speaks up from this centered place and relaxes into knowing she belongs.

The aim here is to proactively change our body's conditioning. By deliberately shifting from tension to ease and center, we can access our wisdom and speak and act from this inner strength. Orienting from a somatic sense of center produces a kind of strength and authenticity that builds trust and respect with others. For those of us with physical challenges, this practice calms the mind and body and steadies emotions.

Cultivating Embodied Wisdom

Working with Richard and Desda, centering practices, meditation, and managing my own energy sensing became routine. Over time these new practices enabled me to feel more ease, clarity, and joy. I invite you to experiment with these suggestions to learn what works for you.

Start by paying attention to your joy as a signal of how to increase aliveness. Become committed to fostering more of what energizes you. Become an observer of your body language. What is your body telling you about this situation or that option? Is the narrative that is embodied supportive of your aspirations? Or is it limiting your capacity to grow?

Notice others as their bodies reveal their moods and attitudes. Trust that your body has in fact accumulated much wisdom, and part of your work is to discern what it is telling you and whether this is useful or getting in the way of living. As you relinquish your compensating strategies—trying hard, in my case—you allow your wisdom to surface. The positive core deep within comes forth more fully as you make space for this.

PRACTICE

> To develop this, practice listening to your experience in silence. Start by sitting quietly for 5 or 10 minutes in a comfortable and upright posture. Plant your feet solidly on the floor below you, shoulders down and back,

> eyes closed and spine erect, and take a few deep breaths from your belly. Then notice your breathing either as it enters through your nostrils or as your chest rises and then falls. Start at the crown of your head and slowly place attention on what you are experiencing as you mentally travel throughout your torso, limbs, and feet, noticing how you feel from the inside.

As we move from feeling the adverse aspects of our disability or life challenge we also recognize our strengths. I struggled with being sensitive all my life. I felt it was a problem. As my vision deteriorated, my hearing became much more attuned to the subtlest sounds. My body became sensitive to foods as a result of a sensitive gut and a prolonged dose of antibiotics.

Frankly, I saw this all as weakness and vulnerability. I tried hard to shield myself and overcompensate, pushing myself to be something I was not. As I began to let go of these ways of thinking and habits, I saw the many gifts in my developing sensitivities. Through somatic practices I became more centered and grounded, and these sensitivities sprouted into gifts.

Finding ground enabled me to explore the light side of my body's wisdom, a deep and rich intuition. Your sensitivities may point to unclaimed gifts. Take steps to deepen and strengthen the gifts which are emerging.

Discern the differences between old patterns that contract your life energy and subtle but clear direction emanating from your wisest self. When you notice your body bracing, contracting, or tensing, get curious about what is happening. Distinguish whether this tightness signals healthy warning signs or some old conditioning which repeatedly puts you unnecessarily into a stress response.

Develop a way to interpret what your body is telling you. Practice embodying resilience by moving toward what you care about with a centered presence.

QUESTION

What is your body telling you about your experience right now?

PRACTICE

Stop and listen for at least five minutes to what is happening in your mind and body. Listen to the breath as an anchor. Notice what emerges.

CHAPTER 6

NAVIGATING FROM WITHIN

"The intuitive mind is a sacred gift and the rational mind is a faithful servant. We have created a society that honors the servant and has forgotten the gift."
—Attributed to Albert Einstein

In the last chapter we explored how to create a grounded embodiment from which we can begin to access our internal wisdom. In this chapter we'll delve deeper into accessing that wisdom within. Learning to trust our intuitive voice is central to navigating through life with integrity, no matter what challenges we face in mind, body, or spirit. As you experiment with your internal compass as I did, you will learn how to decipher your own wisdom.

Uncertainty and doubt lessen as we operate from this inner strength. By cultivating our intuitive gifts, navigating becomes easier. Choices become clear, as does discerning when to say "yes" and "no." For those facing illness or physical challenges, developing shortcuts to our inner guidance enables us to worry less and be more comfortable with our decisions.

Now that I'm more aware and in touch with my body's wisdom, I begin experimenting with it. A friend and I wander into a new age gift shop together. The shop is full of an otherworldly air. A magical universe exists inside the multitude of crystals, meditation bells, jewelry, books, and statues. The sweet fragrance of spiritual scents wafts through the air.

The book section beckons to me. I peruse the titles, fondly recognizing authors such as Louise Hay. Slowly a mood of gentle optimism washes over me. The setting reminds me of that period in my life when metaphysical thinking and writings were at the forefront of my mind. I happen upon a display with decks of cards. I immediately wonder if my friend Tracy would enjoy one. I identify two decks that may be a fit for her, and am uncertain which one to choose.

I casually ask the sales clerk if she has any experience with either deck. I tell her I'm trying to make up my mind about which deck would be best for my friend. She says that I can ask my body which deck to purchase. She instructs me to hold each deck up in front of my solar plexus and inwardly ask, "Is this the best deck to give to my friend?" She suggests that my body will give me a sign, perhaps moving forward slightly for "yes" and moving backward slightly to indicate "no."

While I think the idea is a little hokey, I decide to try it. As I hold the first deck, asking the question inwardly, I notice my torso and body above my feet gently pull forward. I am amazed. I put that deck down and repeat the exercise with the second one. My body moves slightly backward. I try it again and get the same results.

My curiosity is piqued. I find myself at health food stores asking my body which supplement or food is best for my health. I have become intolerant of many foods—wheat, soy, and dairy among them. My vision impairment makes it hard, if not impossible, to read labels, so I alternate between asking a storekeeper to read the labels for me and querying my body.

I find it difficult to calibrate the answers my body is giving me. Sometimes I get a green light on a new snack item, for example, that turns out to be a bad choice for my stomach. I wonder why. It comes to me that I may be asking a large-scale measuring instrument to weigh an infinitesimal item. Sort of like going to a truck weigh station along the interstate after lunch to check my weight. I become curious about how and when to consult this newly discovered resource. Perhaps there is a "Rosetta stone" within me that can decipher this new inner language.

I also notice a wider variation in my body's responses. Sometimes my core will swivel around on my hips, as if I'm dancing with a hula hoop. That move seems to indicate positivity and joy. I keep experimenting and noticing the results. By the time I consider becoming an apprentice in the CoreIndividuation training program, I've developed some amount of trust and predictability with this process. When I ask whether or not to apply for the program, I have multiple body "yes" responses.

Toward Authenticity and Wholeness

Throughout apprentice training, I witness healing and growth. Emotionally, my prevailing mood lightens. The negative charges with the "friction points" in my relationships diffuse. It's as if the circuits of these long-held wounds are severed or discharged. Physically, I feel consistently more grounded and "in my body." Energy and sensation awaken in me. Mentally, my awareness of both my inner and outer experiences has sharpened. Spiritually, the intuitive awareness I have developed astounds me.

I observe healing with clients as well. For a highly intuitive client, our work centers on strengthening her "energetic container." She was so sensitive to external stimulation and the weather systems of those around her that she needed to fortify her boundaries.

In one healing session, she expressed exasperation at her default behavior of taking care of others and ignoring her own needs. Her clarity came to life as she described interactions in her family, work life, and personal relationships.

Acting as the responsible caregiver in her family living across the country, she worried about the well-being of her parents. She felt engulfed in her near obsession with a man who seemed distant and unpredictable. Her natural care for others shone through in her role as a health care provider. She declares that she is ready to stop compulsively giving so much.

We zero in on a particular set of beliefs that are limiting her choices in relationships. She remembers at a young age feeling solely responsible for her family's well-being. At that time, she concluded that their safety was up to her. She carried this core belief—"It's all up to me"—into her adult life.

While she enjoyed the many benefits of believing this—independence, strength, a sense of responsibility, a strong work ethic—there were also costs. She felt out of balance in these relationships, lacking a sense of mutual care and attention. Together we released the energetic hold these beliefs had lodged within her.

This enables her to function from a centeredness she had not known before. It's as if she has transformed her way of being from that of a young sapling, vulnerable to wind and the elements, to a mature oak tree with deep roots.

After years of seeing the power of this work, over and over again I see how those who commit to a regimen of CoreIndividuation healing become steady and grounded. Clients deepen their resilience and intuition.

A client who has anger issues in intimate relationships identifies strong patterns in her family that are also present in her marriage. She feels herself falling into the angry outbursts reminiscent of her father, or slipping into avoidance and minimizing patterns similar to her mother's behaviors. We unravel an energetic dynamic in her body that was locking these patterns in, and the energetic release opens up the possibility for new ways of being.

For a client who is days away from open heart surgery, we clear a congestion in her heart chakra.[1] She reports feeling less armored, more open to receiving the love from her family members. Rather than finding fault with them, she experiences gratitude and love as her husband and son express caring before and after her surgery.

Healing the Subtle Energy Anatomy

Why and how does CoreIndividuation work? I will highlight a few of the organizing principles. Consult Desda's website www.yoursacredanatomy.com for more in-depth explanations.

What we know is that the human body possesses stellar intelligence. The complex inner workings of this organism and its systems to fight off disease and restore homeostasis are multi-dimensional. Both ancient and modern healing techniques point to the sheer wonder of this amazing network of neurons and cells that organize around health and healing.

This same wonder and mystery arises with energy. Energy at a scientific level has many observable properties. It shifts and changes, produces heat, and transforms molecules from one state to another.

The energy within and surrounding our bodies also shapes our felt sense and experiences. When we are alone in a room, and a living being enters, we notice. We even notice the "energetic imprint" of the being. We sense without perhaps knowing why when someone is predatory in nature. We contract and shore up our energy. We walk into a room or a store and feel a difference immediately as the "energy" shapes our experiences. We notice these subtleties when we are present and not floating in the oblivion of our thoughts.

We have a relationship with our energy-sensing capability even when we haven't explored it. Deep empathy for someone we love, sensing someone around us, feeling the different "energy fields" of places and of different groups are all signals sent from our energetic sensors.

Of course, there are neurons within our brains and molecules throughout our bodies that sense these subtle distinctions. Mirror neurons resonate as we sense another's experience as our own. I suspect these mirror neurons work in tandem with our primary energetic sensing organ and energetic nervous system, the template, with hundreds of sensing tendrils capturing data from all around us. The minute I begin a phone conversation with a healing client, I start to feel shifts in my mood, body, and mental framework, which predictably show up in our work together.

Again and again, I witness the intention for a client's human energy structure to be clear and move toward wholeness. I see in myself an impulse toward healing. I'm not talking about the inner compulsion to fix or eradicate disease or darkness.

The gentle and slow healing across decades that I've experienced seems softly held or guided by something greater than myself. My experience is gradual awakening, growth, and wholeness. No doubt this is not everyone's path or experience. I see it with clients who are willing to face and move through difficulties, past their pain to the freedom and joy that lies just beyond.

Frequently clients arrive for our meetings with a flurry of energy, speaking in a somewhat anxious or unfocused way. When clients show up in this state, I ask them where their attention and focus is located. If they are busily fixating on another person's issue or problem, or trying to figure something out and spinning while doing so, I speculate that they are living "from the neck up." Once centered, the clarity and wisdom shows up for the coaching conversation.

Fine-Tuning Our Instrument

During a training called "Awakening the Nine Levels of Sensing" in which we explore our felt sense and awareness, I deepen my ways of sensing.

Two experiences stand out for me in this week. We are nestled in the Berkshires in a retreat center dedicated solely to our group. Each day we explore another level of sensing. One day, I experience a deep sense of rejection in a group dynamic. I feel as if I've been run over by an emotional Mack Truck.

Regina, our co-facilitator, witnesses this and meets me as I head for the door. I think I could walk barefoot in the woods for hours in deep rage and anger. She beckons me to pause, asserting that I have what in CoreIndividuation is called a "life pattern" that is ripe for healing. It is only through my trust in our relationship that I can maintain connection and do the healing work. We work through and release the life pattern, and I'm relieved.

This experience reinforces the new way I'm coming to see difficult emotional territory. Strong triggering instances are the earmarks of a need for release and healing work and the possibility of transformation.

In class we are exploring our awareness of others' physical well-being. We have a guest join us for the medical intuitive portion of our work. She sits in the middle of a circle surrounded by class participants. I return to the class once the guest has arrived and instructions have been shared with the class about how to sense into her physical body.

Each person is asked to sense a different part of her anatomy. I'm assigned to sense her feet and ankles. Aware that I have not benefited from full instruction, I suspect that I won't perceive her anatomy. We are guided through a process and asked to focus in on what we are seeing inwardly in our assigned areas.

In my mind's eye I see the feet, which amazes me. I zero in and see a big red bubble around one of her big toes. I sense other images, symbols in a language I haven't yet studied. When it comes time to share what we've sensed, the experiences are varied, yet focused. Most folks share at least one piece of information that resonates with the guest. When I share what I sensed, she smiles and says she had stubbed her big toe that morning on a table leg.

Toward the end of the weeklong course, we take a nighttime stroll through the woods, up to a point atop a nearby hill. There is a weeded path with branches above and rocks underfoot. We carry flashlights to illuminate the darkened path. There is a gentle chill in the summer air around us. As we begin the ascent, Regina offers her arm so we can navigate together up the dark and pebbled path.

My inner sense of peace and calm accompanies me on the journey. I could be feeling anxious about getting snagged in low-lying branches or roots beneath my feet, but anxiety is absent from my inner landscape. I rely on Regina and my own internal compass to navigate the long climb.

Regina and I develop a rhythm and resonance as we stride together up the dark path. We arrive at the brilliant campfire and I notice Regina's eyes are closed. I ask her about this, and she says she wanted to experience my world of vision loss and deepen her inner sight. She relied on her own inner capacities in solidarity with me.

These examples reveal ways of knowing and sensing that as yet are unexplored. The inner conversation of doubt about what I sense shifts to one of gratitude. Without fully understanding *how* I sensed, I'm beginning to trust that I can.

Inner Sight

What is vision, then, when one can see at these levels? Is it to ascertain reality? Is it to see "what is" and "what is possible"? Is it to see wholeness where there is brokenness? Is it about seeing beyond what is readily observable?

Vision seems to me to be a multi-dimensional process. As it receives data and transmissions from a multitude of sources, vision synthesizes these into whole fabric. Not exclusively the domain of physical sight, vision is a sifting through inputs with discernment. This creative process takes time and concentration. It requires a willingness to "see differently" or with a wide aperture.

There is a not knowing, a curiosity that accompanies this process as well. It's seeing the puzzle put together and not put together at the same time. It requires holding possibilities alive while anchoring what we do know.

I think one way in which my vision impairment has helped me to see is that with 20/20 vision, it is so easy to assume we are seeing the whole picture. This certainty may reduce rather than expand curiosity and possibility. When I'm coaching on the phone, I often close my eyes so that all of my capacities can listen and bring up images and possibilities.

Living from Inner Wisdom

As I continue to build a relationship with these "ways of awareness," I experiment with their use in my daily life. For years I have uttered in prayer, "Show me the way." Sometimes a synchronicity would point to an answer or next step. Two or three people would refer to the same book or article within a short span of time. I would tell myself, "This is a sign, a next step." Participating in this universal school of learning richly affirms the trust I hold in God, myself, and in life. Although this simplistic theology for living may not answer all life's burning questions, it is practical when one is in the flow.

The distinctions around inner clarity I have been witnessing simply deepen this trust. I decide in 2009 to humor the inner wisdom I am receiving by honoring it. This experiment at its core is about understanding and building a relationship with this inner wisdom. My infinitely practical set of questions focuses on how to live more fully and spiritually.

I track inner guidance in response to prayers and inner inquiries, as well as unsolicited direction. I receive subtle inner promptings about what to do in a given relationship, whether to make a particular commitment, or even how to spend my time and energy. The guidance focuses primarily on me rather than others: what I might do or say in a situation, how I might move or take action, or what is happening that I might not realize.

For example, I tend to chew on relationship dynamics until I no longer have any clarity about what is the best course for me. I will hear something like, "There is no problem here." I take this to mean that all my inner gnashing of teeth is for naught. It helps to refocus my mind to think that maybe there is no real problem for me to figure out.

I will hear something like "Be with yourself," and remember to focus my attention on my own direct experience. I hear "Don't worry" frequently and it reminds me of the standard biblical angel line, "Be not afraid."

My learning includes truly digesting the wisdom, not just at a cognitive level, but deep within my bones. If I only marginally absorb what I hear, the depth and impact evaporates rather quickly. Even a simple message like "Be with yourself" can shift me toward a whole set of next steps, including befriending myself and my experiences. Early on I tended to hear these sometimes profound messages at a very pedestrian level, continuing down my own path without an intention to absorb the messages.

The other very practical example is that I ask for guidance on actual directions. Bear in mind, this is imperfect. I can no longer read the signs in the subway system pointing to the various train lines. When I get off at a metro stop that is a transfer station with multiple lines, I will ask for inner guidance. *Which way now?*

Sometimes I will receive clarity without particularly hearing anything. I will know to take a right or a left, go up the escalator, or down the stairs. More often, I will receive a word or phrase; "Right here," for example. I do not hear a voice with any personal qualities, but nonetheless the words connect to my question and feel like an answer. I don't plan on rolling the dice in Vegas anytime soon, and recognize there is much territory to explore.

Theology of Imminence

In the Education for Ministry program I attended, we considered scholarly explorations about the nature of God. This discussion examined the theology of a God who is both omnipotent and omnipresent. Classic theological tension exists between the notion of a God who is everywhere all the time and all-powerful.

If omnipotence and omnipresence coexist, the classic theodicy question emerges, "Why does God let bad things happen?"[2] My personal application of these age-old questions goes something like this: "If I am being led by some wise inner voice, or the God inside of me, why do bad things still happen to me?"

For one thing, I see this as a major collapsing in of my own expectations and understandings. Who said the spiritual life was exempt from loss, grief, and the myriad of emotional ups and downs we all face? For another, I regularly forget to query this inner wisdom about this or that. But it does raise the question of role.

Perhaps this inner wisdom is a support that one engages to learn from life rather than to keep making the same mistakes. I still learn, and grow, and fall short as a human being at times. I still feel angst about long-standing unresolved issues and suffer my own garden-variety anxieties.

I feel genuinely grateful for the guidance, which is often profound. I know that it comes forth from a different stream than my routine patterns of thinking. The quality of the guidance is God-centered, peaceful, and wise. Whether it causes me to look at the big picture, or have more compassion, or set clear boundaries, I appreciate the help. The more I listen, and honor what I hear, the clearer the wisdom.

For so long, I doubted my own inner dialogue. In part it was an issue of discernment. I had impulses that I did not trust or value and inner criticism which drained me. There were also fears that appeared so solid and certain, coupled with insecurities that dangled in the mix of voices, shedding doubt on all clarity that emerged. This patchwork of personalities nearly overshadowed this subtle yet still voice of clarity.

Early in the apprentice training, I compared my sensing capability to others. Classmates would see and sense things I could not perceive. Then I was encouraged to hone my own gifts and stop rejecting them.

I share my budding relationship with my inner wisdom with very few people. I find the level of clarity and specificity I receive to be mysterious, if not suspicious. I have grown so accustomed to floundering around while in the midst of making a decision that I assume there is a very long lag time between my prayers and God's answers. I suspect I am just not on God's top list of priorities, and never really assumed I had a built-in mechanism of my own for wisdom and discernment. I doubt the clarity because it seems oddly immediate.

I have two friends with whom I share my learning journey around intuition. These conversations are precious and private, sneak-away moments in which I disclose my wonder and questions. I become more confident about my inner clarity through each conversation and the support I receive from my CoreIndividuation colleagues

One evening I am walking the labyrinth at the National Cathedral. Once a month two cloth labyrinths are set up for use by those who wish to explore their spirituality in this way. This ancient mystical practice is best approached in silence—following the circular path of the labyrinth like one would approach a meditation.

One foot, then another, movement without attention to getting to a destination, allowing the path to guide one's feet through the journey. I am struck by the possibility of truly allowing the path to be the object of focus, just like in a meditation.

Then it occurs to me: my work is to follow my own path. That's it. Listening for and honoring my own guidance system is simpler than I'd ever thought. Instead of trying so hard to figure things out, my intuition, like the labyrinth, guides me toward my next step.

Learning to Trust Your Body Wisdom

The idea that our intuition is a legitimate aspect of our nature paves the way for a trusted relationship with this inner wisdom. As we begin to cultivate this trust, we gain access to a level of authentic wisdom that guides us.

Committed listening is essential for cultivating this inner relationship. Whether it is a pause, or inhalation which beckons inner wisdom, or a journaling regimen, dedication is integral. Creating a meditation practice and quiet zones within our day fosters our capacity to discern the various voices within.

My encounters and experimentation with intuition still live in the world of mystery. I marvel at my deepening awareness, and am wary of defining my growing capacity. For as clearly as I hear inner wisdom, much remains unknown. What would enhance my understanding of the guidance I receive? Does it matter how I phrase my questions or prayers? Was this a gift that resulted from my vision loss? Or did the vision loss motivate me to listen more deeply and to build an inner navigation system that replaced my physical sight? Mostly these curiosities glide around in my mind like fish in a pristine pool of gratitude as I luxuriate in the learning.

I invite you to consider the possibility that you can sharpen the relationship you have with your own inner wisdom. This intuitive resource can help you to live even more effectively and wisely. At the very least, this inner wisdom may alleviate some anxiety you experience as a result of your challenges when you learn to rely on your inner compass.

Become an explorer of what and how you sense. Suspend judgment as you pay attention to your body, your experiences of the unseen yet sensed, and ideas that seem to arrive out of nowhere. Become deeply curious about how this is working in your life.

QUESTIONS

What is your inner sense of clarity like? How do you experience and recognize the still, small voice within?

PRACTICE

> Set an intention to cultivate your relationship with your wisdom in a particular arena of your life. Stay with the inquiry that unfolds without being attached to getting t right.

CHAPTER 7

LIVING FROM THE CORE

"You can't repress the presence of your soul and not pay a price for it."

—John O'Donohue

Until the last few years when I learned to live from my core, my primary way of being in the world was to try hard. I studied hard to get As and Bs. In college, I was one of those people who went to the library to study, not just to socialize. There's earnestness in the kind of dedication I have had in my life, a commitment toward career and results.

I won an award in my thirties for my dedication on the job. I was the kind of employee who worked hard first, then sought acknowledgment or recognition. I might think of myself as a martyr at times, feeling defeated if I didn't receive acknowledgment for having almost wiped myself out on some project or effort.

Coping with gradual vision loss has only exacerbated this work ethic. I felt at the firm that if folks found out about my low vision, I would not be chosen for projects. I didn't want clients to complain or feel like I took longer than other consultants to get things done or I wouldn't be put on projects. In that system, this was real, not just my fear. I was actually told this by one manager. So I made a decision somewhere in all of this that I had to redouble my efforts and prove myself even more than before, so I wouldn't be overlooked. I'm what they call a try-hard person.

This wasn't just on the job; it was in relationships too. The analogy I heard was that if a relationship were like a tennis match, one does not need to jump over the net and hit the ball back to oneself, but wait for the ball to travel back before hitting it again. I was one of those people who jumped over the net and hit the ball back to myself, in terms of thinking a relationship was all up to me. Sounds pretty exhausting, doesn't it? I'm feeling tired just writing this.

Since then, I've experimented with practices that shift my attention, raise my awareness, or cause me to let go, so I can shift from pushing so hard in life to operating from my core with ease, flow, and joy. I've uncovered long-held assumptions about the way the world works, about my part in it, about support and asking for help. I've plunged into new arenas and new emotions, and declared that I was a learner and a novice when it came to trusting and allowing life to unfold.

These beliefs around striving and pushing hard in life change through my healing experience. Working to clear the human energy structure expands my perspectives on leadership, as well as spiritual and personal development. I see how important it is to clear ourselves and align with our own energy. As a result of the CoreIndividuation work, I feel emotionally lighter and more focused. It's like a calm is jelling inwardly and being expressed without conscious thought. My fellow healers also demonstrate a growing sense of authenticity, and clients seem to be in greater alignment with their life energy. We are all asking, "How do we cultivate our inner core of brilliance?"

In this chapter, we will deepen this inquiry. We'll explore how intentional practices clear the "energetic debris" we accumulate and learn what energizes and refuels our spirit and soul. You'll explore how to manage your own energy. Imagine creating a sustainable and fuel-efficient way of living that reenergizes you and keeps you thriving. Building on your awareness of your experiences and greater alignment with your sense of purpose, you'll explore how you manage and rekindle your inner spark of aliveness. Creating energy sustainability is essential for thriving.

From my CoreIndividuation work, here is what I have come to understand. Energy emanates from a waterfall-like source deep within our center. It's a vital force of light and clarity, like the filament in a lightbulb. Located at the physical center of our bodies and incorporating the spine, this brilliant stream of energy is called the core and reaches from 10 to 20 feet above our heads to 10 to 20 feet below our feet. Imagine a surging yet contained column of energy coming down and through your center that acts as an energy foundation. The chakras, or energy centers, intersect this grand column of energy.

Practice

> Take a moment to investigate this core. Center as you learned to do in chapter five. Stand with your feet hip-distance apart, solidly anchoring into the floor below as if you were a mountain. Now imagine this core of energy from top to bottom, starting approximately 10–20 feet above your head and tracking your felt sense all the way to the other end, located 10–20 feet below your feet. Visualize a triple-current stream—blue, red, golden yellow—pulsate and stream through your body and beyond. Pause if you lose the connection and visualize it again. Once you've regained it, continue to track it to the bottom of your human energy structure.

Just as we absorb and cling to negative thoughts and difficult feelings, our human energy structures hold debris. Before I understood this conceptually,

I had a sense of it in my life. After a difficult business meeting, or facilitating a conflict for a team, for instance, I felt drained. Or extended time with an extremely negative person felt like soaking in a gritty pool, which left me thirsty for space and alone time.

Once I began studying CoreIndividuation, I cleared my own energetic structure as needed. When my mood became negative and a sense of heaviness settled in, it was time to clear. I also became curious about how to tend to my energetic structure. I pondered which experiences enhanced my energetic vitality and which did not. Being in nature almost always restored my energy and clarity.

I became mindful of folding more of the enlivening activities into my days, and managing how much of the draining activities were part of my regimen. My intention to care for my energy and aliveness sprang from a deeper desire to enjoy the flow of life and living. Strengthening my own energetic capacities has proven invaluable in engaging in the world around me.

Here's how you can begin to activate this in your life: Imagine holding an intention to clear away whatever is in the way of living fully and enabling the flow of this brilliant energy. Such an intention might look like this: *I want to live fully, engaging in life without fear or worry dominating my experience. I want to access my own sense of life energy and move from this place of inspiration and possibility.* As you choose again and again to move from your heart's desire, you won't allow your circumstances to encumber you as much.

Taking Ownership for Clearing Inner and Outer Clutter

For each aspect of our well-being, there are practices which declutter and clear our inner and outer worlds. In the physical environment around us, lack of clutter and debris can energize us. Roommates have called me a "piles" person. I do not possess the organizing gene. I buy books on how to organize and lose them. I do what the books say when I find them again. If there were an "Organizing Olympics," the only class I could compete in would be the "most improved." I do know that when accumulated piles clutter my office, there begins to be a place of "stuckness" within me. The only remedy is to pause what I'm doing and declutter, organize, and make the space around me clear.

The vitality and focus that comes to me after one of these cleaning spurts is remarkable. It's as if my mind cannot focus with so much clutter around me.

Just as it is in our physical space, in our spiritual well-being, clearing is beneficial. I am only able to hold so much inner resentment and judgment before I become bogged down. Low-lying negativity takes its toll on my mood and outlook. I need to pause and clear these, through journaling, meditation, and prayer.

I think I have a built-in spiritual toxicity meter which signals when I've sloughed off my spiritual practices. Perhaps this is my conscience. Although I don't impose my own spiritual regime on clients, I do ask them to be accountable for the growth and depth of their spirit.

We accumulate narratives and beliefs that form the foundation of our thinking and attitudes. We rely on this bedrock to assess situations and people, make decisions, and plan for our future. We may not know that some of these beliefs are founded on fault lines within our own perceptions. We often don't realize how much these narratives shape our experiences and our seeing.

Disciplining ourselves to "see through" our stories, or engage others to help us do this, is essential for growth. Stories that limit our power, choices, and possibilities often correspond to moods of resignation and despair. Developing an ambitious practice of uncovering and clearing these narratives keeps life rich and fresh for learning.

Freeing up these stories also brings new light to the emotions that undergird them. Emotions are often the gateway that reveals areas of potential for growth and release. For example, for years I've felt the pain of not belonging. I can fall into harboring resentments for not being invited or included in groups, comparing myself to others who seem to be in the inner circle, and pushing people away when the feelings are too painful. The pattern may be reinforced by circumstances around me, but the beliefs and narratives are definitely my felt patterns.

I decide one day I want to heal this within me and stop trying to change others. I uncovered the story of "otherness" underneath the feelings—that I don't fit in, that I am not worthy to belong. This is a common story for those of us who have some physical impairment, although we are by no means the only ones who can get caught up in it.

I befriend the disappointment and anger that accompanies this story. I ask others who thrive in groups for insights about building community. I ask for feedback from those I trust on how I contribute to this exclusion dynamic that keeps playing out in my life. I see how much I expect others in groups or communities to make me feel wanted and cared for.

I begin to tend to my own needs for feeling valued and cared for and step back from the communities where this need was sorely wanting. I discern where to place my own attention in relationships. With my expectations in check, I shift into a posture of generosity as I approach new groups. I experiment with asking for what I want more explicitly than before. I develop friendships with individuals in communities rather than waiting for others to initiate connection. I recognize that others also have feelings similar to mine.

Energy and Relationships

Several CoreIndividuation procedures also work in clearing dynamics between two or more people. When each person airs and owns their part in a difficulty, it lessens the negative charge between two people and makes new conversations and actions possible. Before my CoreIndividuation training, I could feel these dynamics both in myself and with others, so it made sense to learn that the negative charge between people was not just emotional and cognitive, but energetic as well.

For instance, a client engages me to support her in shifting how she shows up with her husband. She describes her inability to handle angry feelings. She explains her patterns of selfishness and guilt for past infidelity. Her goal is to be a loving wife and handle her difficult emotions skillfully. But the web of negative emotions and narrative encumbers her openness in this significant relationship.

During our first session she elaborates on the tense dynamics between her and her husband. I sense a strong fragrance of shame, guilt, and dominance waft over me as I listen. It sounds like the automatic dance the couple falls into leaves my client feeling ashamed, guilty, and beneath her husband. The feelings have a heavy, locked-in quality to them.

Energetically, the two have merged in a way that isn't useful and doesn't allow her the space to embody her full wisdom. We clear this. She feels a lightness as the pressure in her chest dissipates. She reports later that the shift is quite palpable for both of them. A sense of buoyancy and joy returns to their interactions. They are able to hold an extended intimate conversation in which he reports that she is open, calm, and not defended. The healing work we did enabled her to shift so that she could be herself.

When you find yourself obsessing about another person, take a minute to center yourself. Stand and feel your feet, your belly, and your full length. Imagine your brilliant human energy structure. Concentrate on the field of energy around you as you reconnect with your wholeness. From this place, think about your deepest intention for yourself and the other person. Then act from that place.

Clearing Group Energy

It's also possible to clear energy within a group. During the CoreIndividuation apprentice training, we form close bonds in our learning cohort. As we approach a transition from one year of study to the next, Desda sets aside time for the group to clear whatever "debris" has accumulated before moving to the next level.

We are invited to "clean up" any lingering residue and speak from the heart if truths have been withheld or appreciations have gone unexpressed. We take time to speak to classmates to clear away lingering negativity and give thanks where due. We allow space for all these conversations to be completed. It is as if the group cannot transition to the next energetic level of learning until this clearing occurs.

Clearing the group dynamic illuminated the shared life of the group. Whether individuals saw this group as a class they were simply attending or a "team" devoted to creating healing in the world, Desda held that we created a shared "vibration." By perceiving our group this way, we became intentional and responsible for stewarding our shared work. This made me more acutely attentive to the emotional, psychological, and spiritual wellness of teams. If team members tend to their shared life, the "sacredness" or "vibration" bears the fruits of their efforts.

Living from Vitality

In the 1990s I attended a series of Landmark courses.[1] Despite my ambivalence about requests to enroll others in courses, I learned important life lessons from this curriculum. The one that stands out came from the "Vitality Seminar," which promised to increase one's sense of aliveness. Each week we were given the same assignment: throw a party and invite as many people as you can.

I remember vividly how I contracted inside when I heard those instructions each week. I would lean over to a classmate and utter some version of, "UGH! Here we go again!" I could feel myself recoil at the thought of reaching out to friends and colleagues in an inviting, engaging manner. This tapped directly into my vulnerabilities around being rejected. Taking on this assignment demanded that I feel that vulnerability freshly each week, and move through it.

Another assignment was to clear up our resentments and make space for our relationships to be rekindled or revived. Putting the two assignments together, I held a dinner party and made it a point to invite those people I had "mentally annihilated" because of some mildewed resentment that was gathering dust. This select group of people had earned their rightful place with a chip on my shoulder, and I thought it might clear the air for me to invite them to this party.

Making phone calls to extend the invitation shifted my outdated negativity toward each person. Of course, I did not tell them why they had received my special invitation. That was my own secret experiment. My true intention was to bulldoze through my worn-out, lingering negative stories and to reconnect to my appreciation for whom these people had been in my life.

Saturday evening rolled around, and I had a group of eight or so friends, many of whom I'd fallen out of touch with for months. One by one they arrived, and we embraced and reconnected. It was an unusually warm December evening, so warm that I suggested we eat at the picnic table in the courtyard behind my building. We carried our plates and drinks out to the backyard and settled in.

There was a giddiness and light-heartedness that arose among the group. We laughed and told stories about old times. We celebrated the history we had shared together. We became so exuberant that a neighbor from an adjoining building leaned out her window and told us to quiet down. I was thrilled with this experiment. What a way to break through my lingering negativity!

Who would think that moving through my fears and vulnerabilities would clear the way for aliveness? This practice of continuing to move toward my heart's aliveness became pivotal for increasing my vitality. Now, every time I recognize a pocket of resentment, heavy judgment, negativity or fear, it becomes a target for transformation. The loss of my vision accentuates all of these feelings. In talking with those who experience severe physical challenges, I realize I'm not alone. Such feelings are a natural response to continual loss.

As I commit to living and moving through resentments, fears, and insecurities, I now explore my motives when I put off some action. Am I avoiding something out of a sense of insecurity, afraid I won't be validated? Am I stalling because I'm afraid of something else, some inner doubt or reservation? Am I avoiding action because my motives feel too mixed, with fear or resentment diluting my sense of clarity about taking this step? What wisdom is held in this fear of moving forward? Or is inertia my primary obstacle?

While on a weeklong meditation retreat it came to me that virtually every move I have made arose out of some anxiety. Fear of something happening or not happening was present deep at the core of my being. It didn't seem to matter that much what my mind fixated on or worried about. Although there were some recurring concerns, mostly I noticed how much anxiety pervaded my interior landscape.

I begin to explore ways to temper this underlying anxiety by moving toward joy. Sure, I might push myself out the door for a brisk early morning walk to maintain my health, but I can connect with joy as my legs move along the path, noting each breath, feeling the cool air brush my cheeks.

Later at a trade show for blind and visually impaired persons, I meet a blind man while mingling near a booth. I'm grumbling over some frustration or another as I open our conversation. He says, "One of the problems with vision loss is that if you're not careful, your world will get smaller and smaller. Finally, you will have built a prison for yourself." He encourages me to consciously move beyond the challenges that threaten to keep my life small.

Negotiating vision loss in a fully-sighted world, managing transportation as a non-driver, seeking connection and opportunity to learn and grow require moving beyond discomfort. Seeing discomfort as a reason to avoid or put off some life-expanding opportunity only makes it harder to take on the challenge the next time. The adage "Inaction breeds fear" rings true for me here.

While it's prudent to consider our limitations, organizing our entire lives around them may corrode our spirit. It's a dance of living with very real barriers without unnecessarily limiting ourselves. I needed to clear a lot of fear before I could "dance" most effectively.

What is true for you? Is what's holding you back a real limitation in your circumstances or some kind of pattern of old stuckness that no longer serves you? Where do you need to challenge yourself to embrace more of your vitality?

There's a kind of courage that arises when you face the unobstructed truth of a situation and open yourself to possibility. Once the energy to move through a barrier or challenge shows up, you can engage the hero or heroine within and commit to reestablishing dignity in each new encounter. You know that just beneath your skin, fear and anxiety linger. But you also know that each time you meet your challenge head-on, a certain momentum takes shape and increases your sense of aliveness.

The trick is to rekindle our life energy through taking risks and moving beyond inaction while being present for our experiences. Paradoxically, if I push through a challenge from a "try hard" place, I increase the risk of energetical or emotional bruises. It's not sustainable for me to simply drive hard through challenges, because in those moments I'm not paying attention to my experience.

Every time I search out a new venue I expose myself to the anxiety of getting lost, as I am unable to see addresses or read street signs. I use a smartphone app called "Where the Hell Am I?" to discern nearby addresses, and I frequently ask strangers for directions. Once I arrive at the new destination I'm delighted that I didn't allow my momentary discomfort to stop me from making the trip.

Seeing What Really Matters

I take a break from work to walk in the nearby zoo. Strolling through the lively scenery on this warm summer day revives me. Kids jumping in and out of water spouts, families gawking at the elephants, and the panda passionately devouring bamboo are among the vivid scenes. On my return route, I notice some flashing lights at the intersection I cross daily. I can't make out what has happened, so I meander home.

A short while later I again step out for a trip to the neighborhood library. As I approach the same intersection, I notice several police cars and a small crowd looking at the scene. I ask someone what has happened. One person points to a pair of bright red shoes situated in the far right lane of the six-lane bridge. She says, "Someone was hit crossing the street, and those are her shoes." Turns out this woman had family visiting from out of town for her birthday, which was the following day. She was struck and killed by a van while crossing with the light.

There is something about the image of the shoes which lingers in my mind. I'd been walking about five minutes behind this woman when she was struck. A tender feeling of vulnerability, perhaps fragility, settles in my chest. I realize how solidly I hold my plans and allow them to serve as proxy for my inner sense of security. I pray for the woman's soul and family, as a way of metabolizing this loss. I cross this and other intersections with trepidation for the next few weeks.

Looking back, the proximity and intimacy of this experience pierced the veil which my habits afford me. Although it produced fragility and sadness in me, it also opened up tenderness as I developed fresh eyes to soak in the world around me.

Short of facing a crisis, I need to find ways to regularly return to what is most important to me. Otherwise, everyday worries and concerns will shape my living. I pass people in the metro station to catch a train and reduce them to obstacles in my way. I see a store clerk as a functionary in my day. My mind devotes its processing capacity to minute challenges like how to structure my errands. Efficiency is important, but is it the very fabric of this quilt I call life?

There is a cost to allowing life's "efficiency trap" to swallow us whole. Whatever complacency arises from checking off all our "to-dos" distorts our sense of true meaning and fulfillment. What I find is that it is never enough. When the game I play in life is to take care of all my pending to-dos and ignore the roses that are planted in my path, emptiness arises once my list is done.

It isn't that getting things done is not important to me. I must recognize the illusion that I spin for myself that getting things done is all there is to life. I give up so much when I enable this pattern to stand in for real living. Sometimes my visual impairment exacerbates this dynamic. I focus on what needs to be done, whether it is trying to meet up with a person in a public space, or trying to find a salesperson in a store. My energy and attention get easily wrapped up in just trying to accomplish what is right in front of me.

While on retreat once at St. Benedict's Monastery in Snowmass, Colorado, I was struck by the ending of the liturgical day. During the last service the monks held before retiring, the abbot's final words each night were, "A peaceful death." I thought, "How morbid!" Why not say, "A blessed night of sleep to all"? I asked him about this. He said it serves as a reminder of the preciousness of life and the quilt of impermanence which holds us. Maybe there is an openness that lives in being awake to life's impermanent nature and tasting the joy of the moment. Steering clear of denying death without running from life—this is the zone I want to live in.

How do we rise above the fog of thinking that details and efficiency constitute a meaningful life? We each possess the capacity to rise above the daily current of life activity and see the big picture. As if surfing the "big wave," we extend beyond the place where we get toppled over by every incoming whitecap. We go deeper so that we can rise above it all. We do this in a crisis. We are naturally drawn to questions of priorities, how we spend our time and the people around us we love. We "bottom line" assess how we're doing at honoring ourselves and our values.

It is perhaps only then that we take comfort in knowing we can "true ourselves" to our own inner compass and redefine what we care most about. This way of seeing affords me the opportunity to "right" the direction and flow of my daily life when necessary. I know for me it's all about love, in the end. Am I contributing to the world's love quotient? Is the love I bring to the work I do touching others to live more fully? Those are the questions I ask to help me come from love. What are yours?

When I get caught up in my "hamster-wheel mind" and lose the perspective that I want to come from love, I find peace in returning to my center. In meditation when snared by spiraling thoughts of worry, I focus on my body sensations. I know I can't gain clarity when my mind is spinning out of control somewhere outside of my body.

I get caught in such a spiral when I worry about the status of a particular relationship. Once I recognize I am spinning, I stand up, ground my awareness, place one hand just below my belly, and center. I feel a solid feeling of being rooted.

Eventually a few simple words percolate up from my center. "Be with yourself." I think to myself, "I'm not asking about me; I want a forecast for this relationship." Then, I let the words resonate throughout my body.

Okay, I get it. Be in the present moment. Orient inwardly, stop trying to solve some problem "out there," and track and be with my own sensations, feelings, and experience. Clarity and direction emerge from this centeredness.

Living from Your Core

Once we stop mindless busy activity, how do we live in such a way that we honor our soul's brilliance? Allow our energy and momentum to guide us in our everyday life. Enrich our days with activities that enliven us—from being in nature, to enjoying music, to expressing our creativity. Get curious about what energizes and drains us. Pay attention to our energy and aliveness and operate as if we are the only person who can navigate on our soul's behalf through life's terrain.

We seek opportunities to generate our vitality through risk taking—building connections, reaching out, creating fun and inspiring adventures. Create a game for ourselves. Can we move through this discomfort to renew our life energy or expand our world? Dignity lives in the place where we face our limitations and we move through challenges while honoring ourselves. The energy we cultivate when we move through perceived challenges helps us thrive.

Press the pause button when you notice you are swept up in trying too hard. Breathe and shift the tempo so you orient from a workable pace. Pull back when you get caught up in the swirl of thinking it's all up to you (or some other perfectionist refrain). Breathe.

As we take time to consider what is most important to us, we realign with what we really care about.

QUESTION

What is one thing worth doing today to enrich your life, even if you encounter obstacles?

PRACTICE

Identify an area of your emotional, physical, mental, or spiritual life in which clearing away outdated or unwanted debris would be useful. Use one of the techniques I suggest in this chapter to release what is getting in the way of thriving.

CHAPTER 8

HONORING YOURSELF AS YOU LEARN

"You have to count on living every single day in a way you believe will make you feel good about your life."

—Jane Seymour

Imagine a world in which what is directly in front of you is blurred. Disability awareness trainers invite the fully-sighted curious-minded to peer through a pair of goggles swabbed with Vaseline to experience central vision loss.

Those with macular degeneration move their head from side to side to capture the details of what is in front of them. We struggle to piece together unfamiliar faces, objects, and scenes. By moving from side to side, the unimpaired parts of the macula capture the detail and patch together a quilted image that is translated by the brain.

Imagine you are walking along a sidewalk when a bicyclist suddenly appears a few feet in front of you. You don't have the benefit of seeing her approach, gauging the speed and tracking the trajectory to anticipate the bike's arrival.

Or imagine that you are at a birthday celebration for a friend or relative. You know there will be people you know at the party, but don't know for sure whom you will see. A good friend approaches you, without speaking, and you introduce yourself. Worse yet, imagine that you have a warm and fuzzy conversation with someone and then while at the hors d'oeuvres table, you introduce yourself to the same person again. Meanwhile, you're trying to make out whether the red and maize-colored appetizers are chips and salsa or fruit. You stand back to see how others approach this platter before diving in. Oh yes, you have food sensitivities, so you'd better be sure before you take a bite.

I walk into a drugstore and ask for assistance. It may take some time just to locate an employee these days. Since I cannot read the overhead signs describing what is in each aisle, I ask. "I'm looking for dental floss," I remark. The person says, "Aisle 10, on the right." I then continue, "I'm visually impaired. Can you show me where the floss is." I hold up my empty floss container.

Or let's say I'm working on a document on the computer. Zoomtext, my screen magnification software, enlarges the font by multiples of two and beyond. I use eight times magnification for most things. I'm working on a Word document, let's say a book, for example. At any given time, with this level of magnification, I can see about one-eighth of the full page. I am constantly enlarging and decreasing the font size so I can maneuver around the document. On a website, I reduce the font size so I can see drop-down boxes or buttons. When buying a plane ticket online, I enter the information and then reduce the font in search of the button to advance the process.

That's the fog in my outer world, but there's also fog in my inner world. I get a call from someone who I look up to. Maybe they bark at me and I feel easily intimidated. Or maybe they play into my guilt feelings, whether they mean to or not. In our conversation they make a request, and some impulsive, people-pleasing, conflict-avoiding part of me steps right over my own sense of self and says yes.

Some part of me notices this all happening and my body contracts and tightens. I wonder, "How did this happen?" I'm busy, I'm overbooked, and I just said yes to this or that. In these moments, their needs trump mine. It doesn't feel at all congruent with my best intentions. It feels completely automatic. This fog is where I forget who I am, what I need and want. I turn on myself and become hateful or mean, withholding, unkind.

No matter what challenge or disability you deal with, you have ways you beat yourself up or are unkind to yourself. This can be particularly true for those of us who have a great deal of accommodating we must do to function in the world. Frankly, life is harder for us and we need soft cushions to land on. It's so easy to fall into self-pity rather than offering ourselves the love and compassion we need when we struggle.

I had to learn practical ways to honor myself as I learn. If you reject yourself because of your physical limitations or for any other reason, you will have tools you can use to soften the edges as you reframe the situation. These practices foster self-love and genuine caring. It is this blanket of self-regard that enables us to thrive and grow. Without genuinely caring for ourselves, we shrink and wilt, just like an unwatered houseplant.

Many years ago I co-facilitated a course on enhancing self-esteem at a recovery shelter for women who had faced hard times. The shelter was among a complex of ministries called N Street Village, which occupied an entire city block in Washington DC. Many of the women were recovering from alcohol or drug addiction, abusive relationships or homelessness.

I asked them to come up with three actions they could take that would show love toward themselves. I suggested that these actions be life-enhancing, not short-term pleasures. I gave the example of a bubble bath. One woman raised her hand, and said, "Honey, there isn't a bath anywhere on this block that we can use!" The women laughed and so did I. Fortunately, they all managed to name at least one simple pleasure they could offer freely to themselves.

When I first heard about the concept of loving myself, I had absolutely no idea what that meant. I nestled into books like *The Woman's Comfort Book* to educate myself.[1] Years later, I still find it a rich and somewhat daunting inquiry. Loving myself calls for attention and care at many levels.

Like the bath example above, there are plenty of healthy ways I can "treat myself" that don't involve consuming calories or spending great sums of money. Taking a 20-minute walk in nature or listening to a book on tape with my feet up are simple pleasures that "fuel" creativity and friendliness toward myself.

For me it is particularly important to weave in such moments *before* I'm drained and cranky. This is so crucial for those of us with physical challenges, because outside circumstances are, in fact, harder. It takes us more time and energy to get around, to shop, and to interact. So we need to make sure we're nurturing ourselves so that we have the emotional and physical stamina to do what we want.

I feel frustrated and sad one day when talking with a friend about one of my life challenges. He listens patiently and seems understanding. Then he asks me if there is something I can do to take care of myself. There is a Whole Foods across the street and after our conversation I stroll through to pick up some grocery items. I glance at the whole body section. I invent a game of finding the soap that smells the yummiest to me. My sense of time expands and my world shifts from errand-running pace to the space and time of simple pleasures. I recall the earlier conversation and buy the soap along with the other groceries.

It amazes me how simple this action is and how my mood shifts. I feel treated and special for under $10. This deliberate pause is enough to shift my mood to one of possibility and a feeling of being special. I realize that sometimes all it takes is a small step in some arena where I feel nurtured to shift my orientation to caring for myself. Taking actions to reinforce a positive sense of self-care refocuses the day. Building in activities that foster a sense of joy is another way to keep me in good emotional condition.

But there are times when life challenges get me down. I often turn toward the negative when navigating difficulties with my vision, a challenging relationship dynamic, or just a mood of self-pity. At such times I can ask myself, "What is the most loving way to take care of myself right now?" This practice blunts the sharp edges of the hurts and disappointments I am experiencing and redirects me toward self-care.

The best actions to take depend on the situation. If I'm feeling lonely, I might go for a walk in the park or call a friend. If I'm fixated on some disappointment, I might play some music I love or call a friend to talk about what is bothering me. If I'm burned out from working too hard, I take more drastic measures, such as getting a massage or a manicure.

Being on Our Own Side

There are more subtle ways in which I forget to honor and love myself. As I described in the previous chapter, I often track other people's unresponsiveness or negativity toward me. Without realizing it, I take on the rejection I experience. Most likely, the perceived rejection is unintentional or benign. But I tell myself that it means I'm not valued, loved, or wanted. It's a little like going out in bad weather that just gets worse, until finally I realize I'm in the midst of a bad storm without raincoat or umbrella.

I have absorbed rejection into my self-image. Rejection becomes self-rejection. This blindness to my own wholeness robs me of joy and equanimity. The sooner I recognize I've looped myself into this pattern again, the better. Because every time I notice what I'm doing and choose to be on my own side, I am charting a new neural pathway and breaking free of the old self-destructive habit.

Here's an example. I invite a friend and her boyfriend for a holiday dinner. Weeks go by until I hear back from her. Her email response sends a mixed message. She is available for dinner, but says she may feel differently if I invite a certain other friend of mine.

My heart sinks as I read the email. I feel judged, rejected, and a bit manipulated. I feel my hopes for community and connection are dashed in this friendship that put conditions on whether she will show up in this way in my life. It throws me back to childhood memories of not being enough, not getting what I wanted and feeling rejected. My throat and chest area become constricted and tight, as if rusted and corroding.

In meditation the following morning, I remember the words of Insight Meditation teacher Gil Fronsdal. In an interview, he asked me if a sad or vulnerable three-year-old child appeared, what would I do? I replied that I would hold the child gently, soothing him or her, offering simple, warm words and presence. I would tend to the child's emotional needs for reassurance and love. I realize I could do this for myself. It means stepping aside from the inner chatter around what my response will be to the friend, how I will deal with this, etc., and tending to the part of me which is bruised and hurting.

As I stay present inwardly to these emotions, I feel cared for, met, and honored. I can step back and see the situation with more perspective. My power is not in figuring out the "right" response to this friend but continuing to be with myself in the midst of it all. As I honor the felt experience, a softening occurs, like sun melting ice and snow on a brisk winter day. An ease and peace takes shape as I put all next steps and mental gyrations aside.

Days later, I receive an apology from the friend. We speak about the exchange and I learn more about what has been going on for her. I'm able to share the impact of her message in a clear yet open way, and to see how I contributed to the complex mix of dynamics in play. We deepen our sense of trust and integrity with each other through this process and enjoy a warm and cozy dinner together.

As this example demonstrates, one of the most profound ways for me to cultivate inner friendliness is through mindfulness meditation, which is sitting for a period of time in silence and focusing on breathing as a way to be in the present moment. Noticing the patterns of mind, opening to sensations in the body, touching into the deeper awareness that is not identified with any particular story creates an intimacy within.

Also called Vipassana meditation, which means "to see clearly," the overidentification with long-held narratives loosens as we experience the ebb and flow of the present moment. By bringing kindness to whatever arises within, we find it easier to handle the cacophony of thoughts and emotions that arise.

Here's another example of how it works for me: After a close friend declines my request for a ride home late one night following a spiritual gathering, the disappointment pierces me like a dagger in my chest. Feelings of distrust, fearing others are not really there for me, and a sense of the fragility of my felt sense of support arise.

During meditation the next day, I inquire more deeply into the feelings and sensations in my chest. A core sense of my vulnerability in life arises and expresses itself as fear that I will not be taken care of. I sit with this sensation, opening to the images and feelings. I start to wonder if this is how others have felt toward me at various points in my life. I also see myself withdrawing from the friend like a child who angrily picks up her toys and vanishes from her playmate. What is this child so afraid of?

In my mind's eye I witness a sense of movement, like fast-moving clouds high in the atmosphere, as if the deep cut is beginning to heal. A sense of stillness follows, as if a new perspective has softened the entire encounter. This hurt feels more like a pinprick than a deep and permanent wound. Being present somehow enables me to hold the moment just as a brief interchange amid a long-held friendship, rather than casting in stone a negative story of this friend whose needs and mine collided that evening.

Another way I reject myself is impatience. With my vision challenge, certain activities can be painstaking—threading a needle, looking for my misplaced glasses, finding something at an unfamiliar grocery store, or locating a new destination. I've discovered workarounds for many such activities, but still there are moments when I feel so impatient with the visual challenge I face.

My impulse is to inwardly "beat up" on myself when facing something that should be easy but is not. I can feel impatient about how long the activity will take me compared to how it used to be. In these moments when I can remember to be on my side, the impatience toward myself shifts toward compassion and even humor.

From Self-pity to Compassion

Through mindfulness meditation, I continue to learn about love and compassion, especially for myself. I marvel at the fragrance of peace that lingers after a long, sitting meditation. Meditation is a chance to aerate my soul. When difficult thoughts or feelings arise, I turn toward them with a non-judging warmth of spirit.

I move into the direct experience of the emotions in my body. When I do this, the thoughts soften. My body relaxes into trusting my way of being. I claim space for kindness and inner acceptance. Every time I meet my own inner difficulties this way, I am resurfacing the highways in my mind.

At times, however, I toggle between self-pity and compassion for myself. Both emotional states share the same stem. I have the thought that something is not as it should be. I feel anger about my circumstances. With self-pity, there is a critical veil that clamps down on the experience, resulting in a sense that I am alone in my suffering. If unchecked, I will string together handpicked experiences that form a tightly knit web of despair. Is this true for you too? With self-pity, hope disappears. My body contracts and my life energy diminishes. There can be a very solid quality to the feeling, a sense of victimhood that seals it closed. I am not drawn to connect, share, or move beyond this place of suffering.

I bump into these situations at a museum, for instance, where I cannot read. When I'm alone and there is no audio-described tour or narrated recording of the exhibit highlights, I miss the details. The name of the painting, the placards describing the exhibit, the labels are all beyond my sight capability. I notice that I am alone, when no apparent accommodation is available.

I can feel excluded, ignored, overlooked, and not worth tending to in those times. I can hear my negative self-talk colluding with the circumstances and telling me my needs are not important and not to complain. My inner critic encourages me to stuff my feelings of frustration and simply ignore my needs.

Buddhist teachings distinguish the difference between pity and compassion. Pity occurs when fear meets pain, and compassion is when love meets pain. Compassion for ourselves has a completely different quality in our mind and body than self-pity. The suffering is legitimate and is acknowledged as real. Dignity and respect accompany compassion for ourselves. We accept and recognize the universality of the suffering.

Recently I attended a Dharma talk by Tara Brach, a teacher with Insight Meditation of Washington and author of *Radical Acceptance*.[2] She suggested moving into difficult emotions with two internal messages: "I'm sorry. I care about you," and "Others feel this way." Experimenting with these helps me to feel more connected as I bring kindness towards myself.

Sharing what I'm feeling also moves me past self-pity to compassion and acceptance. Whether I speak to someone who has the same challenge or not, the key is to connect with another who can respect what I share. If the listening has a quality of spaciousness and sincere caring, I can begin to bring that warmth inward.

I encourage you to explore for yourself the difference between self-pity and compassion. Particularly if you experience physical challenges, self-pity isolates and depresses us. It is so easy to fall into self-pity. It can cut us off from what we most need—connecting with others and truly moving through our grief.

Generosity Toward Ourselves

There are times when I am downright stingy toward myself. I withhold tenderness and even connection time from myself. At a core level, this dynamic emanates from that old internal "not enough" conversation. The pattern takes many forms and seems endemic in our culture. It is as if there were an inner absolutism around "being enough" embedded deep in the soil of our collective psyche.

Whether the message is "I'm not doing enough," "I don't have enough," "I haven't achieved enough," or "those around me aren't enough," the underlying anxiety is the same. The "not enough" message arises in the face of fear and vulnerabilities and can only be met with compassion and presence.

Through meditation, I have the felt experience of "enoughness," which melts this mental chatter. In 2010, I attend a silent retreat for women at Spirit Rock Meditation Center in the hills of Marin County, California. The constant downpour of rain overshadows the week with darkened skies that make me wonder if the sun will ever shine again.

I arrive with a mood that matches the weather, feeling downtrodden and dissatisfied. Nothing is to my liking. Maneuvering through the arrival is tense and disturbing. I have notified the center of my vision impairment and food sensitivities, but I want more care around these concerns than I initially experience. Once I know my way around, I'm independent, but since I cannot read signs well, navigating in a complex of buildings without direction is stressful and taxing.

My nervous system is high-pitched as I gather data like a hawk about what isn't working for me. This narrative builds for the first couple of days. The retreat center has responded to the food sensitive among us by creating a separate "simple table" full of food without any spices, oils, or sauces: plain tofu, plain lettuce, rice, etc. While this is a generous gesture, the fact that I can't usually eat the fragrant and sumptuous food on the buffet only furthers my sense of suffering.

There are additional restrictions. Due to the rain, we're asked not to stroll in the nearby walking trails to avoid possible mudslides. I take notes one day during the Dharma talk with my small personal computer, and am asked to refrain from doing so. I have been interacting with the retreat leader and manager around these and other issues through a series of handwritten notes, since we are maintaining silence. The frustration is building within me. I feel like I'm being squeezed into a small box, being suffocated by rules, denial of pleasures, and no way to air these verbally.

One evening after dinner, I burst into tears as I walk in the rain along the main pathway. The grief and frustration pours out like the rain itself. I have internalized these constraints and rules just as I have been doing in my life. My world has grown small, oriented around others' rules to the point where I am ready to burst.

The people-pleasing, accommodating Midwestern friendly part of me is collapsing under the weight of grief and disenchantment. In reference to my primary relationship, I hear inwardly, "You cannot abdicate your life to anyone." Even if I want to use accommodating as a strategy for getting along in life, I can't abdicate my life to another. It just isn't workable for my soul. I'm like the butterfly that can't stay in the chrysalis one more second.

I take these experiences into meditation all week. Subtly I am hoping the suffering will just go away. The teacher cautions us that when we bring our presence to a particular place of suffering, we cannot do so with the hope that it will immediately disappear. This aversive way of meeting our difficulty will not truly relieve our suffering.

The next 45-minute meditation, some force within me faces my inner walls of constraint, not-enoughness, and feelings of being trapped. This inner kindness possesses an undeniable commitment and compassion. It is as if some strong inner presence were saying to me, and to the suffering I have been sitting with, "You matter. I am here to meet you with a loving presence not just for one meditation, but for as long as you need my attention and kindness."

The mountain-like strength and force of the commitment is palpable. It allows me to witness the feelings and sensations that arise. I recognize that I feel subtly strangled and notice my breath cut off at the chest. These constrictions appear in my mind's eye as a black, iron-like substance spreading throughout the chest and throat area.

I tend to the experience with love and kindness, as if I were sitting with a dear friend in need. As I stay attentive, it slowly shifts. The solid nature becomes more porous, like a dark cloud. The darkness slowly dissipates. The constriction eases. By the end of that meditation, the tightness and inner rigidity of thinking and suffering is gone.

This experience remains a vivid example of the quality of inner presence that is available to each of us if we are willing to be with our suffering with awareness and compassion.

Here's how it works for a client who hires me to help her navigate the waters of her predominantly male work environment full of unsatisfying dynamics. She realizes that she slips into a wave of compulsive helpfulness toward the men she works with, only to feel drained and unappreciated afterward. She is so concerned with impressing them that she loses her sense of self and focus along the way.

We spend time exploring the ways she participates in these frustrating patterns, and the impact it is having on her well-being. We design practices for times when she feels the impulse to lapse into helpfulness. For example, after recognizing the impulse to overdo being helpful, she stops, breathes, and asks herself what she needs in that moment. The practice interrupts her habitual impulse and causes her to turn toward caring for herself. She also learns to center, which puts her in touch with her inner wisdom.

She starts orienting around what is important to her. She declines commitments that she knows will distract her from the work that most enlivens her. She makes requests and speaks up about her accomplishments, which is the norm in her environment. She minimizes the impact of critical colleagues by treating herself with kindness. She distills the value of their comments into bite-sized pieces of feedback she can digest. She comes to honor her own experiences, and listens inwardly with respect and kindness. As a result, she learns just how powerful she can be in her environment. Her own inner warmth and acceptance strengthens her emotional well-being. She cares less about how her colleagues behave and focuses instead on increasing her fulfillment at work.

Being Kind to Yourself

Find ways to be truly kind to yourself, particularly when the world is not offering this to you. Access the power of seeing yourself through your own loving and compassionate eyes. Distinguish times of external rejection or disappointment from your own self-perceptions, making space for you to see yourself as whole.

Steward your emotional and spiritual well-being. Cultivate friendliness toward yourself through regular practices such as mindfulness meditation. Generate a sense of dignity when you shift from self-pity to compassion for yourself. If you cannot access inner kindness in such moments of self-doubt, reach out to others who can support you.

Pay attention to how your world gets smaller when you honor others' needs, expectations, and wants at the expense of your own. When you genuinely meet your inner difficult emotions with tenderness, they soften. Take note of when this happens. Access the strength of your own inner, kind-hearted soul during times when you need the attention.

Wherever we are, we can learn about how to love ourselves more fully. Become curious about how the way you see shapes your world. Recognize the suffering you create when you see through the lens of fear and doubt. Take ownership of how you see yourself and others.

QUESTION

What is the most loving way for you to take care of yourself right now?

PRACTICE

Do one kind thing for yourself each day.

CHAPTER 9

CONNECTING AUTHENTICALLY WITH OTHERS

"Life doesn't make any sense without interdependence. We need each other, and the sooner we learn that, the better for us all."

—Erik Erikson

So much of my transition from the fully-sighted world to the low-vision one has been shaped by the many interactions with others along the way. Just as I have been adjusting to the progressive stages of sight loss, so the ways I connect with others have adapted. Given that for the first two decades of my life I was fully sighted, I'm still learning how to interact with others and include my vision challenges. How we disclose and bring our disability or life challenge into relationships is so personal. For me it comes down to intention. I want to be real with others and connect with dignity.

It doesn't always feel dignified. I approach the counter at a fast food restaurant and prepare to ask for help. Aware of the quick pace at which orders are typically placed at the register, I feel anxious. How can I make clear that I need help without completely disrupting the flow of commerce at the counter?

I explain that I'm visually impaired and that I need some assistance placing my order. The cashier looks confused, so I point to my eyes and say I need help. I feel apologetic. The cashier replies, "It's okay, no problem." I cringe. Is he saying it is not a problem that I'm visually impaired? He hands me a printed menu—in a font I cannot read even with my handheld magnifier. Maybe a customer behind me will step in and help.

I feel like I'm causing a problem. My breath shortens as I wonder how to do this. There is temporary confusion, and then all comes to order. The cashier rings up my salad and I pay him. He smiles as he hands me my receipt. I ask what the number on the receipt is so I can claim my lunch when it is called. I feel relieved as I step aside to pick up plastic utensils and a napkin. No wonder one of my low-vision friends avoids negotiating in new surroundings like this restaurant.

Experimentation is the core strategy that keeps me engaged. I try something and see what works. I talk to others who face similar challenges and sometimes those who don't. Most days I'm up for this learning. When I'm not, it's usually because I've become snagged in negative self-talk. Some squeaky little gremlin is tugging at me, telling me I'm causing a fuss, and it's not worth it, or maybe I'm not worth it. The sooner I recognize that this negativity is not the truth, the sooner I can readjust my mindset toward self-honoring.

In close relationships, negative self-talk crops up too. Uncovering and striking down disempowering narratives such as "I can't honor myself in this relationship because I need him or her" enables me to maintain my dignity. At these times I pay attention to honoring myself.

When we experience physical challenges, we often need support from others. In my case, transportation and technical assistance with my computer top my list of needs for support. When something goes wrong with either of these, I experience anxiety and a momentary sense of helplessness. It's crucial to find reliable, competent resources to take care of our needs. When these needs are met by a loved one, the vulnerability and dependence subtly changes the power differential in the relationship.

We can feel intensely tied to another—forgetting that our needs can usually be met independently of the relationship. Getting to a place of true choice about how we want to be in our relationships allows us to act with integrity. As we access the courage and inner strength to live in alignment with our values, we experience our full dignity and aliveness.

What Is Integrity?

WordNet defines integrity as an undivided or unbroken completeness or totality.[1] Wikipedia highlights perceived consistency of actions, values, methods, measures, principles, expectations and outcomes.[2] The *Oxford English Dictionary* says integrity is the condition of having no part or element taken away or wanting; an undivided or unbroken state; material wholeness, completeness, entirety.

Imagine feeling undivided completeness and wholeness—if even just for a moment. I approach this when I am centered and grounded somatically. What gets in my way? Negative stories and beliefs about myself. I take on this negative self-talk when it first arises and dismantle the thoughts, as we discussed in chapter 8. But what do we do when our negativity turns toward others?

For years I've suspected that when I feel strong anger, resentment, or judgment, there is some way I am not seeing clearly. There is a way that my internal case against someone is too solid, too one-sided, for even my own internal justice meter. When I coach someone who is singularly focused on blaming another, laying out how the other person has jeopardized their own sanity, safety, or serenity, I sense internal dissonance. Somewhere this client is unable to access a sense of power.

When I get stuck in seeing someone in this way, I am suffering from emotional myopia. If I blind myself further by profusely complaining about the person, or stockpiling negative anecdotes about things they've done, I drain my own spiritual well. The groundswell of negativity sparks consequences which cause suffering and pain. I'm viscerally triggered whenever they do what I don't like, and my feelings are outwardly observable to others. In these moments I have lost my sense of center.

QUESTIONS

> In her book *Loving What Is,* Byron Katie offers a very targeted and effective approach to shifting these inner conversations and the impact they have in relationships.[3] She suggests taking our particularly aversive relationships and working through a series of four questions. When considering a belief about another person we think has caused us misery, we can ask:
>
> 1. Is this true?
> 2. Can you know that this is absolutely true?
> 3. How do you react when you think that thought? How do you treat yourself/the other person when you have this thought?
> 4. Who would you be without that thought?

I work through this process with my aversive feelings toward a good friend. She has a direct way of making requests in our relationship. When she makes a straightforward request, I feel like a deer caught in the headlights. I experience strong inward pressure to comply with her request, and feel I'm being pushed or cajoled to do something I may not want to do. The feeling usually muddles my clarity to the point that I don't know what I want in the moment. I have started deferring when these direct requests arise, saying I'll get back to her within a stated period of time. But when she asks me to pay for her parking, I find myself just saying yes. I feel pinched and unable to communicate much of anything about this.

The next morning I decide to try the four questions. The thought I'm having is, "I don't trust her when she tries to control me." As I plod through the questions, the emotional charge diffuses. It occurs to me that she may be working on making clear requests. I begin to question whether she is trying to control me or simply making her own needs explicit. The two of us possess subtle style differences in how we make our needs known. Although I might be more comfortable with a different approach, my thinking continues, I am committed to spaciousness and flexibility in relationships.

The Katie approach winds up with what she calls a turnaround in which one completely reverses the core thought. The approach invites us to experiment with various interpretations until one seems even truer than the original statement. The original statement was "I don't trust her when she tries to control me." So I turn the original statement around to "I trust her when she makes a request," and "I don't trust her when I try to control her."

When I create the turnaround "I don't trust myself when she makes a request," I realize I've hit a home run. What this reveals is that there is an underlying internal power imbalance in me. When she makes a request, I feel I cannot say no. While her style may activate my fear sensors, I undervalue my own voice, truth, and power in the situation. I make her right and me wrong.

The shift I am seeking is to truly honor what I want, feel, and need in the moment in this and other relationships. New learning will arise when I meet the "deer in headlights" response to a situation with my own compassion and presence. I can ask myself, "What do I want here?"

Subtly, my mind reasons that because I am visually challenged, I am more dependent on others than most.

It sets up an unhealthy bias against articulating my own needs and wants in relationships. I fight this thought, but it persists. Just as I did when I held onto my jobs in the past, I tend to subtly disregard my needs in relationships. Truly thriving includes tending to the internal messages we are hearing about relationships. As we tease out negative beliefs, we can replace these beliefs with affirming ones which honor our wholeness. Do you have a story about why your own needs are not worth expressing?

One of the particularly seductive sinkholes I get swallowed up in is seeing myself as the victim. It's very easy to do this as a "disabled" person. There's a whole narrative that we engage others in when we see ourselves this way. We move into a discourse of complaining, focusing on the other person's actions or negligence. We all seem to know instinctively how to move in these "Oh, isn't it awful," conversations.

The funny thing is, I always feel worse after identifying myself as the victim. Instead of feeling comforted, I feel as if the ground underneath me is quaking. Identifying as a victim sets me up to hurt the other person with a particular blindness to the impact of my behavior. When I hear internally, "It doesn't matter what I do, I can't win," I am falling into this passive no-win posture. Justification of my actions grounded in victimhood bypasses my conscience and enables behaviors that would otherwise not pass thoughtful scrutiny.

Somewhere in the thought sequence of the victim narrative we assess that we have no power. While there are many things in our lives we do not have power to control or change, we do possess the unique capability to author the stories we tell ourselves. Becoming the victim blocks this sense of power.

In a conversation with a fellow seeker, we explore how to hold healthy boundaries in relationships. At a metaphysical level, I wonder what interpretations I hold about others when it comes to setting boundaries. Are others harmful or unsafe?

My friend, who's an engineer, offers a simple but powerful analogy. In physical science, boundaries need to be upheld by a force such as gravity. He speculates that self-love represents the force within human relationships that upholds healthy boundaries. The more self-love, the clearer we are about the importance of honoring ourselves in relationships. We initiate difficult conversations, speak our truth, and take risks from strength.

Wholeness with Oneself, Then with Others

I find myself asking the question, "What does it mean to have integrity in my relationships?" I come to see that my need for harmony and connection obscures my sight at times. When otherwise glaring red flags or troubling patterns arise, I sometimes gloss over issues. I so want to normalize my relationships that I overlook concerns in the hopes that things will work out. When someone does something that jars or triggers me, I tend toward the stress responses of flight or freeze.

Both of these instincts keep me from being honest about the impact of the person's actions. Speaking up when dissonance arises is a learned skill, one I continue to practice. Disregarding the breadth of my particular experience no doubt served me long ago, but does not support me today.

At the individual level, there's having integrity with our inner reflection process and values and outwardly with our words and actions. At the interpersonal level, there's integrity with shared agreements. In groups or organizations we consider integrity in commitments, roles, goals and boundaries.

The place where our values, actions and words are in alignment represents integrity. Because I know about my accommodating and avoiding pattern in relationships, in order to have integrity with myself, I now check in with a friend when I notice some dissonance after an interaction. I can slow down the action in my retelling and look for places of withholding, minimizing, or normalizing of what happened.

Have I held back from disclosing significant parts of my experience? Am I inwardly downplaying my concerns or simply rejecting them because I think others deal with this all the time as well? If my friend helps me see I've glossed over an important piece of truth, I listen. It may be a truth for me to ingest and contemplate, or one to share directly with the person involved. Discernment around the impact and intent I'm hoping for usually yields clarity around this question.

A highly self-reflective client speaks to me about her significant relationship. She explains that when she and her partner first met years ago, she assumed he would not change one significant aspect of his life for her. As the couple explores moving toward greater commitment, she realizes this belief worries her. It feels like a deal breaker. Initially she ignored her concern because she was afraid of losing the relationship altogether. Finally, however, she decides she needs to air her worry to him.

She apologizes for not being truthful with herself or with him. She feels guilty that her concern might thrust the relationship into peril, but she feels she needs to come clean. Together they navigate through the specifics of her concerns and reach a mutually acceptable solution.

In our work together, she realizes this is a pattern—blurring her truth for fear of losing someone or something. She learns to center and experience a solidness, like roots supporting a mighty oak tree. From this place she has greater clarity and trust in herself and is able to have greater integrity with herself and her partner.

Disclosing

I've hidden my visual challenge at times to avoid feeling vulnerable and I've disclosed my situation at other times to build trust or simply to coordinate more effectively with another. Disclosing my vision impairment is sometimes intentional and at other times is the result of frustration.

Some of my visually impaired friends use a cane in large part to communicate their visual limitations in public contexts. For them, asking for directions seems infinitely more understandable to strangers they encounter at airports or train stations as they use the cane to convey their sight loss.

For those of us with hidden or less apparent disabilities, we experiment with disclosing our differently-abledness. According to an estimate from Britain's National Union of Journalists, up to 70 percent of disabilities are hidden.[4] Since my own vision challenge is not readily apparent to others, I enjoy the freedom to disclose it based on personal choice and preference.

I suppose part of my reticence to disclose my disability to new acquaintances is a protective strategy. I can't control how my disclosure will impact another's opinion of me or how we will interact once they know. I have known acquaintances for months who were shocked when I told them I was legally blind. Usually disclosing my vision loss comes as a surprise to others, as they say I seem to do so well. I cringe when I hear this. I wasn't asking for their feedback. Still, I disclose my vision challenges simply to build authentic connection. This is such a personal choice.

I am working with a colleague who is totally blind. We are working in his office downtown as lunchtime approaches. He phones a favorite food vendor just down the street and orders a gyro sandwich to go. I hear him say, "I'm the blind guy." His matter-of-fact reply to her question, "How will I know you?" startled me. Regardless of how we talk about our disability, disclosing is the first step toward building trust.

There are many within the disabilities community who strive for individual independence in daily life. I think dignity lives in this impulse to navigate on one's own. Breaking not only the stereotype of being "handicapped" but also of being a drain on society is so crucial. It's only when I know independence in a relationship that I can operate with autonomy and make honest choices.

The reality is that the way I've accommodated for my own vision loss includes asking others for help. There's a fine line between needing support and feeling dependent. One thing that helps me is to remember that there are others who can help me if this particular person is not helping me in ways that feel empowering. I listen to my body for signs of entanglement that signal unhealthy dependence.

Trusting Others

I receive a generous invitation from my brother and his wife to join them on a ski trip in Colorado. I'm thrilled, as I have not put boot to binder for over 26 years. Downhill skiing is a casualty of vision impairment. I've written it off as something I will never do again. For years, a good friend encouraged me to consider skiing with a program designed to support people with disabilities to safely participate in winter sports. Somehow, until this invitation, I have not taken steps to say "yes" to this opportunity. I learned to ski at age 8 or so, and have loved it over the years.

I mention to a friend that I am going skiing. He tells me of his eighty-year-old neighbor who skis each year and is totally blind. I ask him if I can speak with her before my trip. A few weeks later, we talk. A lifelong skier raised in Switzerland who lost her vision in the past ten years, she describes how she skis now. She and her instructor are connected using a radio system. He trails behind her, guiding her with his voice. She recalls pausing for a breath next to a group ski class. A student offers her praise, suggesting it must take tremendous courage for her to ski. She replies, "No, it doesn't take courage; it takes trust."

She is pointing to the trust required for the kind of interdependence needed to ski safely with her instructor.

I take her wisdom into my own experience skiing. I embark on the trip west with anticipation and anxiety. High wind conditions prevent the departure of the plane I am scheduled to take from Denver to Aspen. A small group of us waiting at the gate decide to pool funds and hire a shuttle bus to drive the four-plus hours to Aspen.

Upon my arrival, I connect with family and then head to bed. In the morning we gear up and carpool to meet our instructors. My brother and sister-in-law are also taking lessons at Snowmass. My instructor, Sally, works with Challenge Aspen, offering instruction for persons with disabilities.

Once paperwork is taken care of and boots, skis, and bindings are set, we prepare to head out. Sally hands me a florescent green and orange bib to wear over my jacket, with the words "blind athlete" boldly printed on both front and back. We head to the slopes. It's a beautiful day—clear skies and sunny, which also means more contrast for seeing the terrain.

Riding up the chairlift, I look down at the bright green and orange vest marking me as a blind skier. I feel close to tears. Some part of me really hates that I'm in the spotlight because of my visual impairment. It dawns on me that this is another adjustment—skiing is possible, but I will have to do it differently from now on. At the same time, I feel touched by the fact that so many people have supported me to do something I have longed to do for years. Yes, I'm skiing after years of assuming I would not be able to ski.

The first two runs feel awkward, like I'm learning for the first time. No falls, but just a stiffness that lingers. On the third run, something else happens. I remember how much I love to ski. My feet and my legs begin to read the slope and move naturally into a flow. How is this all working?

Since I have some vision, Sally and I agree that I will follow behind her. She tells me that she will track me, and if I stop, she will also stop. I concentrate on the clues available to me—the feel and sound of the snow beneath me, the sense of how the edges of my skis interact with the slope and the way my body balances speed and stability. I keep Sally within my field of vision, but every once in a while I let that go. I can actually make out other skiers, so I'm not worried about running into someone. My body remembers how to ski. Even though the skis are shaped differently now, the sensation of moving down the slope is unforgettable. It's exhilarating to ski again after all these years.

Sally guides me to more difficult slopes once she's confident of my ability to stop and slow down. She coaches me on how to let go of my "vintage skiing style," as she puts it. The new skis turn themselves as long as the weight is placed on the turning leg.

As with most things, I learn surprising parallels for life. It turns out the paradox here is that control is greater when one leans forward into the boots, building speed and momentum. Leaning into the hill actually improves my sense of control. How counterintuitive! Where in my life might that apply?

Sally and I constantly check in. I share what's happening for me, and she uses this as a gauge to help me ski better. I commend her on being such a great coach. She reminds me that by sharing openly and candidly with her what I'm experiencing, our partnership yields a good result.

What is working? Talking with Sally about what it is like for me, taking her guidance based on this and what she is seeing, listening to my legs and feet as they sense the terrain and listening to the edges of the skis as they cut into the snow. Trusting these signals and Sally replaces the vision I've lost and enables me to feel confident gliding down the slopes. When the conditions are more challenging, I use centering to connect to my legs and feel more grounded.

Not only do I feel delighted to be skiing again, but I relish the support of my family. My nephew cheers me on, saying, "You look awesome, Sheri."

Vulnerability and Building Trust

In her book, *Daring Greatly*, Brené Brown describes her research on shame.[5] She identifies 12 categories around which research participants experienced shame. Among the categories, several could apply to those of us with health challenges. These include physical or mental health, money and work, being stereotyped or labeled, and appearance and body image.

Brown suggests that shame prevents us from building connections with others. She tells us that what looks like vulnerability from the inside looks like courage from the outside. Paradoxically, when we take the risk to be vulnerable, we build trust and connection. She suggests that vulnerability is courage in you and inadequacy in me. As I work to hide my inadequacy or fear, I lose out on connecting authentically with you.

Experimenting with disclosing my real self, from a place of wholeness, keeps me connected to myself and others. Sometimes I run into a person who is not empathetic, and cannot seem to connect when I take the risk to share something real about my life experience. Usually, authentic disclosure builds depth in my connections with others. The trick is to tell the truth about my experience without whining too much—which is sometimes unavoidable.

I remember hearing years ago on *Saturday Night Live* that whining was really anger coming through a very tiny hole. Better than not coming out at all! Sometimes that's what raw pain feels and sounds like. When I speak honestly and openly, others respond with empathy and compassion.

QUESTION

How do you connect authentically with others?

PRACTICE

Notice what happens in your body when you have, or lack, integrity.

CHAPTER 10

EXPANDING YOUR APERTURE

"The real voyage of discovery consists not in seeking new landscapes, but in having new eyes."
—Attributed to Marcel Proust

My decades-long inquiry around seeing has opened up many portals for my learning. My yearning for restored physical sight yielded emotional healing as I grew to accept and move beyond the vision loss. This loss spurred my spiritual thirst, which created new sight through contemplation, study, and practice in meditation. My desire to be in alignment not only with my sense of purpose but also with my values cultivated integrity. My quest for fulfillment altered the impact of my relationship with the vision loss.

Gradually as I shift from trying to manage loss and change to allowing life to unfold, healing occurs at levels I didn't foresee. This requires me to crack open a window in my heart and mind which leads to the possibility of seeing differently. All the strategies create a way of being with ourselves that enables growth and healing, and expanding our aperture enables us to see and recognize the shift and growth emotionally and spiritually.

Seeing and Creating Beauty

One summer while on vacation with my family in Nantucket, I play with a set of watercolor paints. I limit my time in direct sunlight because it is damaging to my eyes. So I look for indoor or shaded opportunities to amuse myself while everyone else is at the beach. I have always loved to draw and paint, but have never really considered myself talented enough to explore this interest. My legal blindness makes artistry an even less attractive pursuit. But with long stretches of time available during this vacation, I decide to experiment.

I notice a gaggle of watercolor students perched along the cobblestone streets on my walks to town. I wander into a toy and hobby shop and splurge on some cheap paint and paper while there. I paint scenes of the historic New England beach houses engulfed by the wheat-colored beach grasses as they sway in the ocean breeze. Whale-watching turrets called widow's peaks decorate these early-1700s-style houses. I imagine women peering out from the towers, longingly awaiting the return of their ocean-bound husbands. I become completely enveloped in capturing these scenes on paper for hours at a time. At day's end, as my brother says, I have something to show for my time besides a good tan!

A marvelous synchronicity occurs this same week. An article featuring a Nantucket artist appears in the local newspaper. My brother brings this to my attention because the artist also has juvenile macular degeneration. An artist with visual impairment, oh my!

We arrange a visit to her home at the other end of the island. She has never met anyone else with Stargardt's disease, and receives us with warm and open hospitality. She designs elaborate costumes for children's theater productions. She shows us her studio where several of her magical costumes are on display. As a parting gift, she hands me a signed copy of a children's book which she illustrated.

When I return from that trip I sign up for an oil-painting class at the Corcoran School of Art in Washington DC. Located in a restored 1800s schoolhouse in upper Georgetown, the beginning oil-painting class takes place in a spacious classroom adorned with windows overlooking the park below. The majority of the 25 or so students are seeking a degree in fine arts, and attendance is taken at each class. I speak privately to the teacher, informing her of my visual impairment and mentioning that I am a first-time art student. She graciously affirms my eagerness to learn.

We work on several projects over the course of the term. We apply the French technique, layering several washes of paint over a base coat just as the old masters did. We borrow the backgrounds of our favorite paintings and layer a still life in the foreground.

As students arrive for class, we position ourselves in a scattered circle around the subject for our painting that day. I scramble to be close to the subject so that I can see more fully. My monocle, a handheld telescope used by low-vision individuals, becomes an instrument for capturing the details of the subject. At the end of each class, I delicately stow away my freshly moistened canvas, pack my painting toolbox, and ride mass transit home. The aliveness and joy I feel when painting nourishes my desire to learn. This passion motivates me to find creative ways to work around my practical challenges.

It's as if I were having a love affair with this newly explored passion. Even though my learning curve is steep, I linger in every aspect of this new pastime, from mixing paints to the rush of producing something of beauty. At the end of the semester, I have four or so works of art of which I am actually proud. Having grown up with no formal training, I am amazed at the results. Untested narratives around my lack of creativity crumble as the love of creating pours through me.

As with drawing, with painting I have to unlearn how to see. Rather than capturing what is in my mind when painting a live model, I have to concentrate on the shapes and their relationship to one another. My first impulse when painting a leg is to feel self-conscious because I don't know how to paint a leg. But if I break the figure's leg down into a set of connected shapes, I can be true to what I am actually seeing. This is quite a discipline, but also very liberating.

Seeing and capturing the beauty of the shapes, the lines, the edges and the negative space spark the real work of painting. Teachers point out the multitude of colors in human flesh when painting a figure. There are hues of green, yellow, blue, and lavender which emerge in the model's topography. Portraying curves, depth and shape using complementary colors to accent light and shadow becomes an invigorating adventure.

Painting invites me to live in the inquiry, "What is beautiful?" Just as there is a letting go of what I think I see, there is an exploration of the colors and shapes that illuminate the subject. Texture, light and shadow, color, line and brush stroke are among the artist's magical techniques for magnifying beauty and rhythm. I personally am enamored with the use of light and shadow as well as color.

My love of painting has flourished with many wonderful teachers. I receive affirming words such as, "Others should see the world as you see it!" I realize now that I had avoided enrolling in an art class because I simply did not want to be a beginner. In most of the classes I've taken, students who claimed to be beginners were actually picking painting back up again.

Does wanting to look good get in your way too? Is there something you long to do but the fear of being a beginner is stopping you? Perhaps, like with me, the almost-blind painter, what you long to do takes you into the heart of your so-called limitation. A friend told me of an amazing video of a legless dancer. There is something profound about going toward the very thing that is the problem in your life that is amazingly freeing and exciting.

Getting Stuck in the Process

While painting, there's a place I get to where I just want to put the brush down and zip up my project. I'm amazed at what I've created, and don't want to ruin it. I experience a tightness or contraction which feels like aversion to risk. I want to put a bow around the work and stop jeopardizing what I've created.

Of course, there is an appropriate place to stop painting, when toil and overworking are approaching dangers. This aversion I'm describing, however, is where self-consciousness laced with fear creeps in. This spoiler within raises doubts about my abilities and wants me to settle instead for good enough.

One of my painting teachers once said if you can't risk ruining a painting to make it better, you're not painting fully. Wrangling with these inner voices during the creative process teaches me about life. Staring at a blank canvas at the beginning of a three-hour class can be daunting. All the anxieties flood in as I wonder whether I will remember how to paint again this week. Aside from a prayer, deep breathing and centering inwardly, beginning to paint is the only way to translate the anxiety into creation.

As I work to break free of inner critics, I can come to the place of flow. It's where all around melts except the dance I'm engaging in with the emerging design in front of me. Starting with a blank canvas and allowing creation to unfold is exhilarating and emotional work. This is why I paint.

There is an aliveness that painting evokes in me. From the frustrations and points of not knowing what to do next, to the joy of returning to the flow once again, the engagement compels me to be fully present. The passion for beauty is at the sweet spot of this process. Seeing beauty stirs me deeply, enlivening my soul somehow. I find art and design to be such wonderfully healing and soul-compelling aspects of what it is to be fully human.

Handling anxiety is part of the dance. Almost always I thoroughly reject my painting in the process. It takes sheer discipline to continue. Moving from the playful mind of possibility to the evaluating mind disrupts the flow. When I shift toward judging, I see the imperfections rather than the possibilities. My vision becomes reductive as I evaluate and critique mid-process. I ask myself, "How is this turning out?" UGH. I think it is too this or that, etc. Once I metabolize the disappointment, I slowly reengage until I lose myself again in the dance.

When I immerse myself in painting for three hours, I literally see differently. Invariably on the ride home from a painting class I marvel at the colors. The sky, the trees shout out with color, shape, and depth. I notice beauty as if I've been given new eyes. There's something in deepening one's noticing which transforms seeing. An apple becomes a sumptuous shape, with drama portrayed by light and shadow and a luscious mix of alizarin crimson and yellow ochre. My thirst for juice arises as the apple comes to life. I do not know whether beauty emerges or I discover it.

Seeing beauty in patterns, movement, healing, coaching, learning—all exhilarate my senses. There's a transformation that arises when my relationship with the expression or creation of beauty comes alive. Connecting with beauty changes my relationship with what I'm seeing. My creative spirit awakens my sense of aliveness.

Seeing the beauty in another person's path is also energizing for me. Whether it's from disenchantment to empowerment or from resentment to freedom, I can't help but be inspired by the journeys of those I've met as a coach. I marvel as others glimpse who they want to be as they meet the fragility and shadows which encumber their life force. They face a hundred small rounds in the ring of living life to the fullest, each time vanquishing inner and outer villains. They embrace risk and uncertainty as they move toward an ideal yet unrealized future. Creating and moving toward inner dreams and visions is another way we engage our creativity.

For example, a woman engages me because she wants to make a career transition. Trained as an artist, she works in administration with a large organization. She feels she is not fully expressing her true gifts and talents. She speaks about her desire to make a living as an artist, but she cannot really imagine this becoming a reality. She says that even the way she portrays herself shifts when she changes from artist to administrator.

Her hair is naturally curly, with wisps and twists curling around her face. While at her office job, she wears her hair pulled back or straightened. We work with this living metaphor of embodying her authentic nature. Gradually she takes steps toward establishing her own art business. At times she has very little belief that she can make a living as an artist, but she moves toward her internal image of her future. She takes steps to make this happen, and begins to fully embody what she really cares about. Eventually, she becomes a full-time artist working with public art projects, teaching and employing other artists. Her clarity and focus resulted in a major career transition. She exhibited courage and conviction as she moved toward creating her future.

Where does vision come from? When I work with a client to shape their future, there is an impulse, an image, or a mood of excitement that shows up. This urge to expand and grow has been incubating in him or her, stirring both heart and soul. I witness this when I coach. I track a client's energy and aliveness, and listen for what wants to spring forth. I see part of my work as a coach to serve as a midwife to these emergent murmurings of the heart and soul.

Honoring the Unseen

Another way we expand our aperture is by recognizing and paying attention to the unseen. Working with energy has opened my eyes to the unseen yet sensed. I used to think my physical vision loss constrained my sight, but I'm not so sure about that anymore. This journey of macular degeneration has opened as many doors as it has closed. They are doors I probably would never have opened were it not for the loss of my physical sight.

Looking back, I recognize that I have been living in an inquiry all these years: "What does it mean for me to see clearly?" With less than 10 percent of the vision most people take for granted, I have been learning how to cultivate sight from within. By clearing my filters, perspective, and inner lens, my vision is being transformed.

Granting authority to the unseen is a part of this journey. During my CoreIndividuation training, I faced inner doubt and a discrediting of my own inner sense of things. What was a hunch, or my imagination, with experience has become more real in my mind. I recognize that I may have granted too much authority to sources that seemed quite legitimate to me at one time. As my sense of wholeness clarifies, I grant less authority to the negative inner dialogue which creeps in and snares me. Once I recognize the fear that fuels this negativity, it evaporates.

Seeing from the Heart

In our interactions with others, we can practice how we see. When I manage to access my wisest self in the midst of a difficult conversation, a fresh way of seeing opens up. For me this shift toward compassion is pure grace. I'm doing my active listening thing while under my skin I'm jangled like a squirrel racing frenetically to nowhere.

I take a deep breath, or just notice my breath for a moment. I connect with a distant thought about my intentions toward honoring wholeness both in myself and with others. A quiet awareness within me portrays this person I am facing as soft and hurting just under the stream of words. *It must be difficult,* the voice is suggesting. I get how she or he feels because I have felt that way. I empathize. Ouch. I ask inwardly, "What is it like for this person right now?"

When I do this, whatever comes out of my mouth has soaked in the waters of this awareness. Even though I may strain to uphold a sense of being "right," this awareness beckons me to soften and open.

Healing and Gratitude

At a weekly Insight Meditation class, Tara Brach talks about noticing what is happening at any given moment and how we're being with it. Am I avoiding or pushing away my inner experiences? Am I meeting my experiences with kindness and openness? Am I befriending my inner world or rejecting it? Through these questions I see that over the years I have come to a different relationship with my chronic eye disease and my sight loss.

When I finally absorbed the realities of my eye condition, I shifted into a strong commitment to restore my sight. There was a quality of fighting or opposing my disease which in many ways served me. This resilient spirit motivated me to explore alternative therapies, and as I championed the possibility of reversing an incurable disease, my spirit gained strength and momentum.

But there is also an addictive quality in wanting suffering to go away. The restlessness and dissonance which emerges when things are not as I want them to be prevents me from living at peace. Being okay with what is produces acceptance and ease. Perhaps a sense of acceptance emerges like the sunset in the arduous arc of moving through grief and loss. As I accept the abundance and wholeness of my life just as it is, I am freed of the need to change my sight. Ironically this makes me more open for whatever healing occurs.

I speak with a priest about my repeated prayers for vision. I wonder aloud about how my lack of physical healing impacts my faith. I recognize that God is not like a vending machine in terms of answering prayers. Yet some part of me still believes that if I'm sincere in my desires when praying, and I allow that I do not have the bigger picture, somehow I will feel like God is with me. The priest replies, "How do you know your prayers are not being answered?" Maybe my vision has healed, just not in the way I wanted it to.

A Healing Quest

In September 2010, I embark on a healing pilgrimage to New York. Through friends I become familiar with John of God, the internationally recognized Brazilian healer. The last week in September John of God creates space for healing at the Omega Institute in Rhinebeck, New York. Omega retreat participants and nearby commuters come together to witness and experience healing.

Not really knowing what most needs healing, I craft a list of intentions for the week. Right under inner peace I place my physical sight squarely in the queue. While awaiting the train to New York, a deluge of anxieties floods my mind. I fear my vision will not improve as a result of the healing. I desire restored physical sight and yet live in fear that healing won't occur. The vulnerability in seeking healing accompanies the path of unknown but longed-for outcomes.

There's the heavy weight of traditional medicine imposing its prognosis on my future. It's hard to truly maintain a posture of openness while living out the sentence of incurability. The temptation is to sink into doubt as "reality" beckons me into the net of fear. My eye condition is termed incurable for a reason, right? Who am I to think healing can occur?

I call a fellow CoreIndividuation practitioner before boarding the train to give voice to these anxieties. She reminds me that the healing is already bubbling to the surface. These fears and anxieties uncoil as I approach the possibility of change. I inwardly meet the discomfort I am experiencing and affirm my intention to heal.

Once on the train, I share my thoughts with a fellow pilgrim returning to see John of God. She describes anguish while facing breast cancer shortly after giving birth. While I do not hear the story of a medical miracle, her presence is calm and joyful. This calmness rubs off on me with the click-clack of the train rolling toward New York. I melt into the comfort of my seat with renewed openness about the week ahead.

Once settled in at Omega, my anxieties give way to anticipation. Monday morning arrives and some 1,400 of us gather in a white tent on the Omega lawn. All dressed in white as part of the suggested protocol, this wave of white somehow equalizes us in our collective desire for healing. I have brought a photograph of a friend and stand in line to pray for her healing.

From the moment I enter the tent, a sense of light seeps in. I am touched to see so many people intent on healing. Throughout the week, fears, insecurities, and difficult emotions arise. The John of God staff encourage us to pray, "Reveal to me that which needs healing, and show me what I am meant to do to heal."

Immediately after the first "spiritual intervention," I'm overcome by doubt. This is all a hoax, I think. My eyes do not spontaneously heal. I tread water in waves of sadness and a sense of discouragement. For whatever faith and trust I have been able to muster, I expected immediate evidence of transformation.

As part of the suggested healing protocol, I sequester myself in my dorm room, with eyes closed much of the time, sleeping and meditating for the next day. I encounter my share of inner demons. Doubt, fear, insecurity all bubble to the surface.

The John of God staff suggest that the healing first addresses root causes of disease and illness, rather than the physical symptoms. I deduce that these root causes are emotional and spiritual at their core. The need to forgive permeates the messages we receive.

I return to John of God for two more spiritual interventions that week. When coming to the momentary exchange with him, you may make a specific request for healing. I pointed to my eyes on my initial meeting. As I approach him on my third meeting, the words "inner peace" spontaneously spring from my mouth.

I spend most of the week sequestered back in my tiny dorm room napping, praying, and listening inwardly. My inner voice and wisdom become clearer and clearer. I receive many wise nuggets of guidance. Ultimately in this inwardly active journey I encounter a quiet sense of peace and calm. I surrender my intentions to heal over to the mystery of this healing work as trust emerges.

While my vision seems slightly improved, I experience many other shifts. I become aware of changes I want to make in my primary relationship. The year that follows yields one courageous move after another in my life. My prayer life is reinvigorated, I begin a deep meditation practice and my inner voice becomes much clearer. While visiting an eye clinic, I am told my acuity is much better than my records indicate. Shortly after this, a low-vision specialist assesses my acuity and finds it has actually worsened.

I return to Omega to see John of God in 2011. We are led through a forgiveness meditation in which we release lingering resentments. Each time I release another resentment, my body quivers just as it does when I'm doing healing work.

As I sit in the meditation room, awaiting the call to approach John of God, I fall into a clear stream of prayer and meditation. My body begins to rock from side to side, completely involuntarily. I am in some kind of spiritual groove enveloped by joy. Upon approaching John of God, the joy and love electrifies me. During the healing, tears of joy stream down my cheeks. I am so clear in the moment that this joy and peace is the true healing. Looking back on this experience, I'd say someone pressed the "reset" button on my underlying mood.

Finding Peace

Even though my physical sight is unchanged, I am at peace. My perspective about my vision shifts. Joy is my predominant mood. I trust life more than I used to. Love seems at the center of my world more and more often. My inner voice is clearer and is shaping the fabric of my life. It's as if the circumstances in my life were the same, but I'm not the same.

I used to dread the inevitable disappointments in life, and at low moments, wonder whether a light would shine in on the seemingly difficult circumstances. Whether I would pray, call a friend, read some spiritual literature, or get out of my own world and reach out to support others, I never seemed to trust that the prevailing mood would shift. My faith muscles had not stretched beyond the good times to provide much of a safety net during difficulties. But some little piece of light always shone in.

I used to think of this glimmer of light or hope as just a thread, that the true universe was dark and dangerous but God extended a mere thread to lighten the load at just the right time. A friend would call or some true kindness would seep through my pores from another human being. Once again, I was just spared by mere chance from drowning in the well of sadness or despair. Can you relate to this?

Our attention eventually drifts toward some lightness, some beauty, or some spaciousness which opens the door to a new way of seeing. Then we look back and almost forget the terrors of that dark room and the lack of light which we experienced. We go for a walk, we clean the kitchen, we laugh at something unexpected, or our heart opens when we see a child fall and skin her knee. We move beyond the difficult mood as the drift of our humanity sweeps us into another way of being.

But then one day I saw it just like the negative space in a painting. This background space is created by the outlines of the subject of a painting and is harder for most of us to actually notice. Maybe I had it backward. Maybe most of the time I was completely oblivious to the many small miracles, grace, acts of kindness and general abundance that was so much a part of my life I didn't see it.

In subsequent John of God healing episodes, I gain clarity about the long-held question, "What did I not want to see?" I did not want to see myself, the sense of my self as unlovable and broken. Through deep meditation, these perceptions transform through love and compassion. Once again, my physical sight spurs learning at the emotional and spiritual level.

I periodically feel a swell of gratitude for what and how I see. I recognize not everyone feels the kind of peace, compassion, and joy that have come to be the norm for me. I'm so grateful that I see both possibility and light in those whom I work with and befriend. When difficult emotions or narratives arise, I metabolize them more quickly than before. I experience a strong core of centeredness and love that holds me during such times.

Pure joy arises when I see beauty around me. When I get the chance to be of service to another, my inner light expands. As Einstein said, "The most important decision we make is whether we believe we live in a friendly or hostile universe." Maybe my unique way of seeing is the true miracle.

QUESTION

How could I see differently right now?

PRACTICE

Take a few minutes each night before you turn in to capture moments of gratitude. Whether you write in a gratitude journal or in an electronic document as I do, take time to feel the gratitude as you capture specific items for which you are truly grateful.

Notes

Introduction

1. Elyn R. Saks, "Successful and Schizophrenic," *New York Times*, January 25, 2013, accessed March 19, 2014, http://www.nytimes.com/2013/01/27/opinion/sunday/schizophrenic-not-stupid.html.
2. Elyn R. Saks, *The Center Cannot Hold: My Journey Through Madness* (New York: Hyperion, 2007).

Chapter 1: Being with Your Experience

1. For more on Elisabeth Kübler-Ross and the stages of grief, see http://www.businessballs.com/elisabeth_kubler_ross_five_stages_of_grief.htm#elisabeth_kubler-ross_five_stages_of_grief, accessed March 19, 2014.
2. Elisabeth Kübler-Ross, *On Death and Dying* (New York: Scribner, 1997).
3. There have been several studies on the value of light restriction for treating patients with retinal degenerative diseases such as Stargardt's. One May 2006 study on "Light and Inherited Retinal Degeneration" in the *British Journal of Ophthalmology* by D. M. Paskowitz, M. M. LaVail, and J. L. Duncan is available in full at http://bjo.bmj.com/content/90/8/1060.full. (Accessed March 19, 2014. *Br J Ophthalmol* 2006;90:1060-1066 doi:10.1136/bjo.2006.097436.)

Chapter 2: Seeing Your Wholeness

1. Richard N. Bolles, *What Color Is Your Parachute? 2014: A Practical Manual for Job-Hunters and Career-Changers* (New York: Ten Speed Press, 2013). This is the most recent edition of this book, which often appears annually.
2. A Course in Miracles is a self-study curriculum that aims to assist its readers in achieving spiritual transformation. Wikipedia, http://en.wikipedia.org/wiki/A_Course_in_Miracles.
3. Ebenezer Scrooge is the main character of Charles Dickens' 1843 novel, *A Christmas Carol*. By Christmas morning, he's ready to drastically change his life.

Chapter 3: Accessing Dignity

1. Retinitis pigmentosa: Any of several hereditary progressive degenerative diseases of the eye marked by night blindness in the early stages, atrophy and pigment changes in the retina, constriction of the visual field, and eventual blindness.
2. Transcutaneous electrical nerve stimulation (TENS) is the use of electric current produced by a device to stimulate the nerves for therapeutic purposes.
3. Touch for Health is a system of balancing posture, attitude, and life energy to relieve stress aches, and pains, feel and function better, be more effective, clarify and achieve your goals, and enjoy your life. (http://www.touch4health.com/, accessed March 20, 2014.)
4. *The American Heritage Dictionary of the English Language*, 4th edition.
5. The LifeLaunch program is based on the teachings of Frederic M. Hudson. A LifeLaunch is a graduation from one era of your life to another and requires new vision, new plans, and courage as a

person shifts gears. The process is described in Hudson's book, *LifeLaunch: A Passionate Guide to the Rest of Your Life* (Santa Barbara, CA: Hudson Institute Press, 1995).

Chapter 4: Orienting from Purpose

1. Marsha Sinetar, *Do What You Love, the Money Will* Follow*: Discovering Your Right Livelihood* (New York: Dell, 1987).
2. Suzanne G. Farnham, Joseph P. Gill, R. Taylor Mclean, Susan M. Ward, and Parker Palmer, *Listening Hearts: Discerning Call in Community* (Harrisburg, PA: Morehouse Publishing, 1991), 46–47. Used by permission.
3. In a passage that's often quoted and paraphrased, Buechner said that vocation is "where your deep gladness and the world's deep hunger meet." Frederick Buechner, *Wishful Thinking: A Theological ABC* (New York: Harper & Row, 1973), 95.
4. According to a CBS *Moneywatch* report, "More than eight of 10 employees believe that their relationship with their direct supervisor has a big impact on how happy they are with their job." Moreover, surveys show that "the No. 1 reason people leave their jobs is because of their manager." (Suzanne Lucas, "The Top Reason People Leave Their Jobs," CBS *Moneywatch*, October 18, 2013, http://www.cbsnews.com/news/the-top-reason-people-leave-their-jobs/, accessed January 20, 2014.)
5. The Hudson Institute of Santa Barbara characterizes the doldrums as "a down time, a protracted sense of decline, when you're not happy with your life chapter, but you don't think you can do much about it." (http://www.hudsoninstitute.com/pdf/lifelaunch.pdf, page 4, accessed January 20, 2014.)

6. Robert Fritz, *Path of Least Resistance: Learning to Become the Creative Force in Your Own Life* (New York: Ballantine Books, 1989).
7. Martha I. Finney, Deborah Dasch, *Find Your Calling, Love Your Life: Paths to Your Truest Self in Life and Work* (New York: Simon & Schuster, 1998). The quote in the text is from Martha Finney's article "The Career That Calls You" in *Spirit at Work*, October 1998, page 9.

Chapter 5: Cultivating Embodied Wisdom

1. Marguerite Henry, *Misty of Chincoteague* (New York: Rand McNally, 1970).
2. CoreIndividuation is a healing process that has been trademarked by Desda Zuckerman. For more information on the process and its history, see http://desda.com/about/coreindividuation/.
3. For more regarding NFB Newsline, from the National Federation of the Blind, see https://nfo.org/audio-newspaper-service.
4. Craniosacral therapy is a system of gentle touch designed to enhance the functioning of the membranes, tissues, fluids, and bones surrounding or associated with the brain and spinal cord. *Merriam-Webster's 11th Collegiate Dictionary.*
5. The Victor Reader Stream is a handheld media player for the blind and visually impaired. For more information, see http://www.humanware.com/microsite/stream/index.html.

Chapter 6: Navigating from Within

1. Chakra: any of several points of physical or spiritual energy in the human body according to yoga philosophy. *Merriam-Webster's 11th Collegiate Dictionary.*

2. Theodicy, in its most common form, is the attempt to answer the question of why a good God permits the manifestation of evil. Wikipedia, http://en.wikipedia.org/wiki/Theodicy.

Chapter 7: Living from the Core

1. Landmark courses are three-day programs that major on self-help and personal development. For more, see http://www.landmarkworldwide.com/.

Chapter 8: Honoring Yourself as You Learn

1. Jennifer Louden, *The Woman's Comfort Book: A Self-Nurturing Guide for Restoring Balance in Your Life* (San Francisco: HarperOne, 2005).
2. Tara Brach, *Radical Acceptance: Embracing Your Life With the Heart of a Buddha* (New York: Bantam, 2004).

Chapter 9: Connecting Authentically with Others

1. WordNet 3.1, "Integrity," accessed March 31, 2014, wordnetweb.princeton.edu/perl/webwn.
2. Wikipedia, "Integrity," accessed March 31, 2014, http://en.wikipedia.org/wiki/Integrity.
3. Byron Katie, Stephen Mitchell, *Loving What Is: Four Questions That Can Change Your Life* (New York: Three Rivers Press, 2003).
4. Stephen Brookes, Rachel Broady, Lena Calvert, "Hidden Disabilities," National Union of Journalists Disabled Members Council (UK), 2008, accessed April 1, 2014, http://www.disabilityinformationzone.co.uk/pdfs/NationalUnionJournalists/brookes-NUJ-Hidden-disabilities-Report-plus-Lena.pdf.

5. Brené Brown, *Daring Greatly: How the Courage to Be Vulnerable Transforms the Way We Live, Love, Parent, and Lead* (New York: Gotham: 2012).

Resources

For more information about navigating career development, go to www.careercrossroadscoach.com. Check out the blog, which focuses on career renewal, authentic leadership, and managing energy and vitality. For organizations wishing to hire Sheridan as a coach, consultant, or trainer, go to www.purposeatwork.com to learn more about her services.

For more in-depth application of the ten strategies in your own life, go to www.careercrossroadscoach.com, click on the resources page, and enter your email to request *Strategies Into Action*—a guide to each chapter. The guide will help you draw on the book's key themes through a series of questions organized by strategy. These questions will support readers as they reflect on what they've learned and apply these principles in their lives.

Recommended Books

Books have been an integral part of the learning and growing process for me. Below I've listed books that have been significant in helping me cultivate the skills to thrive.

Self-Awareness—Meditation

Ahmaas, A. H. *The Unfolding Now: Realizing Your True Nature Through the Practice of Presence*. Boston: Shambhala, 2008.

Brach, Tara. *Radical Acceptance: Embracing Your Life with the Heart of a Buddha*. New York: Bantam, 2004.

Kabat-Zinn, Jon. *Wherever You Go, There You Are*. New York: Hyperion, 2009.

Kornfield, Jack. *The Wise Heart: A Guide to the Universal Teachings of Buddhist Psychology*. New York: Bantam, 2008.

Transitions and Personal Growth

Bridges, William. *Transitions: Making Sense of Life's Changes*. Expanded and updated. Cambridge, MA: Da Capo Press, 2004.

Brock, Lillie R., and Mary Ann Salerno. *The Change Cycle: The Secret to Getting Through Life's Difficult Changes*. Bridge Builder Media, 1994.

Strozzi-Heckler, Richard. *The Anatomy of Change: A Way to Move Through Life's Transitions*. Berkeley, CA: North Atlantic Books, 1997.

Meaning and Fulfillment

Csikszentmihalyi, Mihaly. *Flow: The Psychology of Optimal Experience: Steps Toward Enhancing the Quality of Life*. New York: Harper and Row, 1990.

Frankl, Viktor E. *Man's Search for Meaning.* Translated by Ilse Lasch. Boston: Beacon Press, 2006.

Cultivating the Positive

Braden, Gregg. *The Spontaneous Healing of Belief: Shattering the Paradigm of False Limits.* Carlsbad, CA: Hay House, 2008.

Lipton, Bruce H. *The Biology of Belief: Unleashing the Power of Consciousness, Matter, & Miracles.* Carlsbad, CA: Hay House, 2013.

Seligman, Martin E. P. *Learned Optimism: How to Change Your Mind and Your Life.* Reprint edition. New York: Vintage Books, 2006.

Spiritual Development

Judith, Anodea. *Eastern Body, Western Mind: Psychology and the Chakra System As a Path to the Self.* Revised edition. New York: Celestial Arts, 2004.

Keating, Thomas. *Open Mind, Open Heart: The Contemplative Dimension of the Gospel.* Amity, 1986.

Myss, Caroline. *Anatomy of the Spirit: The Seven Stages of Power and Healing.* New York: Three Rivers Press, 1996.

Nouwen, Henri. *Life of the Beloved: Spiritual Living in a Secular World.* Tenth Anniversary edition. Crossroad Publishing, 2002.

Palmer, Parker J. *Let Your Life Speak: Listening for the Voice of Vocation.* San Francisco: Jossey-Bass, 1999.

Purpose and Career

Leider, Richard, and David Shapiro. *Whistle While You Work: Heeding Your Life's Calling.* San Francisco: Berrett-Koehler, 2001.

Levoy, Gregg. *Callings: Finding and Following an Authentic Life.* New York: Three Rivers Press, 1997.

Love

Baer, Greg. *Real Love: The Truth About Finding Unconditional Love and Fulfilling Relationships.* Reprint edition. New York: Gotham, 2004.

Stone, Douglas, Bruce Patton, and Sheila Heen. *Difficult Conversations: How to Discuss What Matters Most.* Revised edition. New York: Penguin, 2010.

Williamson, Marianne. *A Return to Love: Reflections on the Principles of "A Course In Miracles."* New York: HarperOne, 1996.

Healing

Bernhard, Toni, and Sylvia Boorstein. *How to Be Sick: A Buddhist-Inspired Guide for the Chronically Ill and Their Caregivers.* Boston: Wisdom Publications, 2010.

Chodron, Pema. *When Things Fall Apart: Heart Advice for Difficult Times.* Reprint edition. Boston: Shambhala, 2000.

Countryman, L. William. *Forgiven and Forgiving.* Harrisburg, PA: Morehouse Publishing, 1998.

Developing Strengths—Overcoming Challenges

Brown, Brené. *Daring Greatly: How the Courage to be Vulnerable Transforms the Way We Live, Love, and Lead.* New York: Gotham: 2012.

Brown, Byron. *Soul Without Shame: A Guide to Liberating Yourself from the Judge Within.* Boston: Shambhala, 1998.

Jeffers, Susan. *Feel the Fear . . . and Do It Anyway: Dynamic Techniques for Turning Fear, Indecision, and Anger Into Power, Action, and Love.* 20th Anniversary edition. New York: Ballantine Books, 2006.

About the Author

Sheridan Gates was diagnosed with a juvenile form of macular degeneration in her early 20s. Since then, she has been searching for the answer to this essential question—"What will enable me to thrive?" She has reinvented her career three times as she forged a path of integration between her professional life, her declining vision, and her budding spirituality.

With over 20 years as a leadership and career coach, Sheridan weaves time-tested strategies for thriving into the needs and concerns of those facing a life challenge that endures. As a leadership and personal development trainer, facilitator, and executive coach, she helps individuals access the power within to achieve the results that matter most to them. Sheridan's clients include leaders, managers and employees in Fortune 500 companies, federal and state government agencies, and nonprofit organizations.

With an MA in Education and Human Development from George Washington University, and a BA in Economics and Business and over 30 years as a business professional, she helps clients integrate the world of performance and success with inner clarity and values. Sheridan is a Professional Certified Coach (PCC), a somatic coach, and a CoreIndividuation practitioner working with individuals committed to a life in which they thrive.

Sheridan serves as faculty and coach for the NTL Institute for Applied Behavioral Science. She serves on the board of the World Institute on Disability.

Sheridan enjoys hiking, painting, meditation, cooking, and travel.

www.ingramcontent.com/pod-product-compliance
Lightning Source LLC
Chambersburg PA
CBHW031600110426
42742CB00036B/505